PUSHING THROUGH THE PAIN

PUSHING THROUGH THE PAIN

Franz Wall

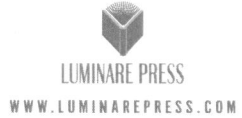

LUMINARE PRESS
WWW.LUMINAREPRESS.COM

Pushing Through the Pain
Copyright © 2025 by Franz Wall

All rights reserved. This book or any portion thereof may not be reproduced or used in any manner whatsoever without the express written permission of the author, except for the use of brief quotations in a book review.

Printed in the United States of America

Luminare Press
442 Charnelton St.
Eugene, OR 97401
www.luminarepress.com

LCCN: 2025920496
ISBN: 979-8-90071-003-7

For those who carried me in ways seen and unseen: through your prayers, your gifts, and your presence, I found the strength to keep pushing forward.

Table of Contents

Introduction | 1

CHAPTER 1
Childhood Dreams | 5

CHAPTER 2
Dental Prep | 19

CHAPTER 3
University of the Pacific | 35

CHAPTER 4
Into the Beyond | 41

CHAPTER 5
Craig Hospital | 55

CHAPTER 6
Learning to Breathe | 63

CHAPTER 7
Daily Life Paralyzed | 73

CHAPTER 8
The Problem of Food | 85

CHAPTER 9
Victory! | 99

CHAPTER 10
An Unlikely Adventure | 107

CHAPTER 11
Palo Alto VA | 111

CHAPTER 12
Mariposa Strong and Home | 123

CHAPTER 13
The Cyst | 133

CHAPTER 14
Through the Darkness | 143

CHAPTER 15
Put Me in Coach! | 155

CHAPTER 16
All for Him | 167

Conclusion | 179

*And I saw the river over which every soul must pass
to reach the kingdom of heaven
and the name of that river was suffering:
and I saw a boat which carries souls across the river
and the name of that boat was love.*

—St. John of the Cross

Introduction

While I don't consider myself an expert on pain and suffering by any means, I have certainly had my fair share of it in the last several years. My suffering is visible to anyone who meets me, but pain wears many faces. Some endure it in silence, carrying invisible wounds the world never notices, while others carry their wounds openly on their body and in their lives for everyone to see. My hope in writing this book is to speak to all who hurt—not with advice too narrowly shaped by my own experience, but with reflections broad enough to meet anyone, anywhere in their journey.

Pain is not something most people want to talk about. It's uncomfortable, messy, and inconvenient—a subject society often tries to erase. In our relentless pursuit of happiness and comfort, we are surrounded by products and messages promising to remove pain, suffering, loss, and regret. Yet genuine healing does not come from avoiding pain, but from walking through it with honesty, faith, and purpose.

The pharmaceutical industry spends billions developing medications that promise quick relief. The self-help industry offers formulas for happiness built on positivity and constant self-improvement. Social media feeds us curated images that hide the struggle behind every smile. These may numb us for a moment, but they cannot erase the truth: pain is an inescapable part of the human story. It is not a flaw in God's design but a place where his grace can do some of its deepest work.

This book is about rejecting the world's impulse to hide from pain and learning instead to push through it—not with empty grit, but with the strength that comes from God. Here you will read about moments from my own journey—the accident that changed everything, the long road of physical rehabilitation, and the hidden battles of the heart and mind. Some of these stories are raw and unfiltered, pulled straight from the days when I wasn't sure I could keep going. Others highlight the breakthroughs—both the dramatic victories and the quiet, unnoticed wins that mattered just as much.

Along the way, I will share the mindset shifts, spiritual lessons, and practical steps that helped me endure. I will be honest about the places I failed, the days I let frustration or pride win, and the ongoing ways God is still refining me. This is not a manual written from the safe distance of hindsight; it is a testimony from the middle of the climb.

My prayer is that as you read, you will see your own reflection in these pages. Our circumstances may be different, but pain is the common ground of humanity. The details of your story will be unique, but the choice we all face is the same: Will we turn away, hide, and try to numb the ache—or will we keep moving forward, trusting that God can redeem what feels unbearable?

This is not only a story about enduring suffering, but about letting it transform you. Each push forward, no matter how small, is not just about reaching your own finish line—it is part of something much bigger. The act of persevering through pain, when united with Christ, carries eternal weight. It shapes your soul for heaven and can touch the lives—even the eternal destinies—of others, in ways you may never see this side of eternity.

By the end of this book, my hope is that you will not only understand the title, *Pushing Through the Pain*, but also embrace it as a personal call to action. That you will see pain not as an interruption to the life you wanted, but as a doorway into the life God intended for you. And that when you turn the final page, you will know—deep in your bones—that every push forward with him is worth it, because it is leading you not just toward recovery or resolution, but toward the salvation of souls and the joy of eternity.

CHAPTER 1

CHILDHOOD DREAMS

I grew up in the small, rural town of Mariposa, California, on a small farm. I was one of nine children, and our days were full of farm work, school, adventures and laughter. We played and fought with equal passion and so learned how to get along in both work and play. Both of my parents are devout Catholics and ensured we were raised with strong religious values.

Growing up in a Catholic household helped instill the principles of my faith from an early age. My parents read us stories of St. Francis, St. Padre Pio, St. Joseph, and so many other saints. These men and women who were so close to God and working miracles always seemed like real-life superheroes. My patron saint is St. Francis, and I would often recite the prayer of St. Francis in the hopes that God would also call me to serve him in a special way. This prayer has been a continual guide and light for me in all that I have done.

> Lord, make me an instrument of your peace:
> where there is hatred, let me sow love;
> where there is injury, pardon;
> where there is doubt, faith;

where there is despair, hope;
where there is darkness, light;
where there is sadness, joy.
O divine Master, grant that I may not so much seek
to be consoled as to console,
to be understood as to understand,
to be loved as to love.
For it is in giving that we receive,
it is in pardoning that we are pardoned,
and it is in dying that we are born to eternal life.

(PRAYER OF ST. FRANCIS)

I wanted to be a hero and a saint. I wanted to be God's instrument in the world and bring about his glory. I prayed that God would give me a clear sign so that I wouldn't have any hesitation in responding to his call. As I had not felt pulled by God in any direction, I resigned myself to pursuing what I loved, knowing that if I wasn't doing what he wanted me to, God would intervene and make his will clear.

Ever since I can remember, I have possessed a driven work ethic and passion for achievement. In school, I applied myself diligently to my studies and consistently earned straight A's. I also excelled in sports, utilizing my natural athletic abilities to help my team achieve victory over the years. Even from a young age, I took great care in mapping out long-term goals and future plans—where I wanted to attend college, what career path I would pursue, and how to optimize my chances for success.

My early education helped nurture independence and self-motivation. For most of grade school, I was home-schooled by my hardworking mother alongside my eight siblings. With so many children to teach, she instilled an appreciation for self-paced learning. I thrived in this environment, easily mastering concepts and taking ownership of my education at an accelerated rate.

By high school, I was enrolled in the local public school so that I could play sports and benefit from more in-depth science classes. The structured learning environment combined well with the habits I had developed through homeschooling, resulting in continued good grades.

At fifteen, my father asked if he could take me out to lunch to discuss my future and what potential careers I was interested in. He told me how he had become interested in law as a young man and with hard work and integrity had eventually become a well-respected deputy of the District Attorney's office. He asked if there was anything I was interested in, or that I could see myself doing. Without hesitation, I told him I had a burning desire to pursue dentistry. I explained how the blend of science, technology, and patient relationships appealed to me. My dad was a little surprised at how quickly I answered his question, and how much I had clearly thought about it. He told me that if I was really interested, he would help me determine the next steps. Together we made a plan. Eager and ambitious as I was, this plan greatly excited me, and I couldn't wait to begin. The first step was graduating from high school and getting into college.

During my junior year of high school, my older brother was preparing his applications for college. The school he wanted to get into was Thomas Aquinas College, a small private Catholic college that taught liberal arts. Since my brother was planning on attending, we sat down as a family and discussed what was needed for the application. As we were going through the prerequisites, I couldn't help but mentally track in my head what I would need to do to apply the following year. However, as we were going through it, one thing stood out to me: The school did not require graduation, only a graduation equivalent, Meaning that I did not have to finish off all four years of high school but could take an exit exam during my junior year and leave a year early. After verifying that my understanding was correct, I signed up to take the California high school proficiency exam and try to skip my senior year. I knew that high school was just a stepping stone to greater things, so if I could shave off a year it would be one year quicker to become a dentist. I had no idea how hard the exit exam would be, but I had to try.

The exam was a couple of months away, and just on the odd chance that I would pass it, I started preparing the rest of my application: asking for letters of recommendation, requesting my transcripts and, of course, taking the SAT. I started putting all the pieces together, and soon enough, I had everything ready to go except for my exam. I was very nervous; I knew that passing this test could mean a whole extra year of my life. I studied hard and went into the exam ready to ace it. When I stepped into the room, I immediately noticed the other students who were taking the exam with me. Most had dyed hair, raggedy clothes, oversized beanies, and many had a glazed look in their eyes. I don't know if they scared me or gave me more confidence that I could pass the test. But I simply put my head down, grabbed the pencil and paper, and began.

Despite being three hours long, the test was over before I knew it. I walked out, feeling semiconfident, but I wouldn't know my scores for a couple of weeks. We began praying and hoping that everything would work out so that I could go to college with my brother. The weeks seemed to drag on, but every time the mail came in, I frantically shuffled through it, looking for a letter from the California Department of Education. The letter finally came. I tore it open, and out of the corner of my eye I saw "Congratulations, you passed!" A great sigh of relief was followed by my family's cheering in celebration.

With the test out of the way, I gathered all of the necessary documents and submitted them, alongside my brother's, to the admissions board at Thomas Aquinas College. Once again, our patience was tested as we waited to hear whether or not we got in. Even with me passing the test, I knew it was a long shot, but that didn't stop me from thinking about it. I was already planning what the next years of my life would look like if I left school early.

Matthew, my older brother, and I came home from school one day, and my family was all standing around the table with excited expressions on their faces. We came into the room at the same time, and there was a telepathic moment of communication when I raised my eyebrows, and an assuming nod came from the family. The letters from college had come with our fates sealed inside, still unopened, so we didn't know, but we were excited to find out. We both looked, and the envelopes were matching in size, so for better or for worse, we knew we were in it together. We tore through the envelopes, and sure enough the first line said, "Congratulations!" I didn't even continue reading. We had been accepted, and were going to college.

Once again, we celebrated, talking about how awesome it was that we could go to school together and be in the same class. We immediately called all of our friends and gave them the good news. It was an exciting time, even though it was just the beginning.

The next day I woke up and went to school just like every other day, but a thought popped into my head. I had taken the California high school proficiency exam, and I had been accepted to Thomas Aquinas College. Did I even need to finish Junior year? Thoughts about getting a job and saving some money, or maybe buying a car, immediately sprung to mind. My mom was gone for a few days visiting her sister, and my dad had already gone to work. Sitting at the kitchen table, I reviewed my situation. It was unique, and I took a minute to appreciate what an opportunity I had in my grasp. Everything seemed to click and add up like a simple math equation, I was already getting into college so why go to school. With a smile, I decided not to go to school that day. Or the next. Or the one after that. I forgot to mention that to my father, who assumed that every day after he left, his children went to school. Suddenly, my mother got a call from the truant officer saying her son had missed school without a note from her. Needless to say, she was furious and drove home, probably yelling at me all the way. The officer explained to us that I needed to give two-weeks' notice, if I was going to leave school. My mom glared at me, and I begrudgingly admitted my mistake. We gave official notice to the school, and as I walked out those doors forever, I let out a sigh of relief. Summer had officially started! It took a while for my classmates to understand what was going on, and I still have some of my old classmates from high school who ask me "What happened to you, man? You just disappeared!"

I wasted no time in getting a job at the local grocery store. While it wasn't glamorous by any means, I enjoyed the work, and it allowed me to earn some extra money before college. The summer came and went with many a last adventure and plenty of memorable moments, all while I was working full time to purchase a car before leaving. I managed to scrape together just enough to make my tuition payment and buy an old beat-up Toyota. When the end of summer finally came, my brother and I packed the car, got the keys, and took off.

Going to Thomas Aquinas College was a life-changing experience. First and foremost, it had a profound effect on my faith. I was born and raised Catholic and always had a strong belief in the faith. But it wasn't until college that I was able to really understand it and prioritize it above everything else in my life. We had the opportunity to read the early Fathers of the Church, and to learn about my faith so that I could explain it in a way that made sense. It was a beautiful thing to read both Aristotle and St. Thomas Aquinas and see how our Catholic Faith was founded on reason. It's easy to believe something, but it's hard to understand it, be able to explain it to others, and stand up for it in the face of the many distractions and adversities in the world.

TAC taught me so much about thinking, and how to have a good discussion. We read the great books, which were directly translated from the original text. We analyzed and discussed them, struggling as a class through any logical inconsistencies. We joined all the philosophers of old in discussing the most important questions of logic, rationality, and man's greater purpose. It is known as the "great conversation," which stretches across all time. Like so many who had gone before us, we compared many philosophies and ideas. The questions posed by the tutors were challenging and yet very rewarding for our class to discuss. Math class taught me how to look at basic principles and build from them using simple logic. Philosophy explored how much our wandering imagination could quickly lead us down the wrong path, as well as how it could be the most powerful tool to discern truth. Science taught me how to learn from experience, building upon the first principles of nature. However, some of the greatest lessons that I learned happened outside of the classroom alongside my peers, growing in the Catholic faith. Being around such strong, like-minded individuals of a similar age, who believed just as earnestly in God and the Catholic faith, reinforced what I already knew to be true and encouraged me to prioritize it in my life above everything else. I have no doubt that one of the big reasons I still have the faith I do today is from those formative years in college and the strength of my family and friends.

College was stressful in many ways. Not only were the classes difficult, but I had the added pressure of knowing I needed to do well to go to a good dental school. This led to many late nights of studying. In addition to this, all of the normal social pressures of relationships, sports, and friendships that came with adjusting to life on campus. However, I made sure I had some fun, I went surfing in the early morning before school. I continued with my wood carving, working out, and enjoyed many philosophical conversations on random topics with my classmates. And so, despite its difficulty, I enjoyed school very much. I learned a lot from my tutors and classmates, and especially from the classwork.

In all this, I always found time to go to the chapel at the end of the day and pray before our Lord. This would always fill my soul with peace, help me put everything into perspective, and give me the strength to continue another day. I also began a special devotion to Mary, often visiting her statue, getting down on my knees, and saying a few Hail

Marys to honor her. I know that my faith is not perfect, but I knew that by asking Mary and our Lord for the strength of perseverance, I would be helped at every point along the way. I also had the opportunity to attend daily Mass, something that I chose to do often. Deep down, I knew there was something special about going to daily Mass, about being close to our Lord, and placing him as a priority above everything else. And while I'm certain I wasted time in many ways at college, the one thing I know for certain is that all of my time spent in Mass was never wasted.

Thankfully, my hard work paid off, and I got top marks across all the subjects during my four years at TAC. As I went through college, I learned a lot about myself and my priorities in life. My goal was to practice dentistry in my small town, and I knew that might mean sacrificing a large salary. While planning my future and looking into options for financing dental school, I realized how expensive it was and what an incredibly large school loan I would end up with. After talking with many dentists, I found that the best option would be to try to get a full-ride scholarship from the military. It was a long shot as only 0.3 percent of applicants earned this scholarship. It was competitive, and I needed not only the best college GPA but a high score on the Dental Aptitude Test and acceptance into dental school. I decided to apply to both the Navy and the Air Force, hoping that I would be selected for a full-ride scholarship. This process would take the next four years, and I knew I would not know the answer till the end, but I knew if I didn't try, I would regret it, so I picked up the phone, called the recruiter, and started the application process.

During my senior year of college, in order to graduate, I was required to write a thesis. The thesis was meant to be a culmination of learning from the four years of the arts. I prayed and thought a lot about what I wanted to write about, and what I wanted to remember and be remembered by. This would be the capstone of my entire four years in college. After a lot of contemplation and self-reflection, I felt drawn toward the idea of the importance of taking care of the human body. I was drawn to the quote from Corinthians: "Do you not know that you are God's temple and that God's Spirit dwells in you?" (1 Corinthians 3:16). I have always felt very strongly that working out and staying fit is important, and that maintaining proper health and taking care of your body is an essential part of living out the faith.

My thesis connected the Old Testament description of the golden temple with the New Testament description of the temple, which is our own body. The Old Testament temple was an intricate building of expensive materials made with specific instructions from God for the sacrifices made to him. In a similar way, our bodies are made by God specifically to be temples of the Holy Spirit, and in their beauty are meant to reflect the beauty of God within. Our bodies are united to Christ's body through the church in a much more intimate way than our relationship to the Old Testament temple. Through these connections we realize the importance of maintaining our bodies so they can reflect the beauty of Christ within us. I explained that this does not mean we must all be bodybuilders or supermodels, but rather that we owe dignity to the body, both by avoiding perverse acts to the body and also by maintaining physical health and fitness. God created us as a union of body and soul, and therefore we must not simply ignore the body and only take care of our soul. We must take care of our body so that it might act as a vessel to carry our soul through this world and into the next.

When contemplating the title for my thesis, I really wanted to title it "I have a Godlike body, a reflection on how our body is a temple of the Holy Spirit." I knew the title would be funny, considering that I was in very good shape at the time, and yet also an extremely direct way to view the point of my thesis. However, I decided against it, thinking it might be a little too immature and instead used "Glorify God in Your Body," which was a more proper and probably more accurate title.

I wrote my thesis and talked with my mom about what it meant to glorify God with our body, and she asked whether or not my thesis only applied to people that were fit and healthy. I explained to her that it did not matter if a body had been beaten down with age or disfigured through multiple pregnancies, it was only a matter of taking care of and preserving the body that God had given us, maintaining its health and proper function, and treating it with respect, dignity, and beauty. The human body, regardless of its condition, is beautiful and ought to be taken care of to the best of our ability.

These words and my thesis may seem at first glance to be ironic. How crazy that I wrote a thesis about having a Godlike body when I was in my prime and as fit as I could be, and yet here I am, in a wheelchair, unable to move 80 percent of my body, reduced to a fraction of strength and capability that I had before. However, my thesis is just as relevant as ever, even more so now than when I wrote it. Because even now, I fight hard to take care of the health and fitness of my body, making the most of its capabilities and treating it with respect, dignity, and beauty. God has chosen my disfigured body to be his temple, and while it might be different from before, it is still my duty to take care of what he has given me.

I urge all of you reading this to take the time to realize the importance of respecting the dignity of your body, to maintain your health and not abuse your body through sinful acts and perverse actions. Maintain your health through exercise and healthy eating while at the same time avoiding harmful and undignified actions. God has only given us one body; we must take care of it.

Graduation came and went with many family members attending. It is always hard, turning a new leaf, saying goodbye to friends and relationships that I knew would never be the same. I wanted to hang onto those friendships that I hoped would last the rest of my life. But now was the time to go forward into the unknown, to strike out and make something of myself. A lot of emotions, thoughts, worries, and excitement came from leaving that college campus, a place that had been my home for the last four years. But I knew I was on the path to something greater, something that I had been preparing for my whole life.

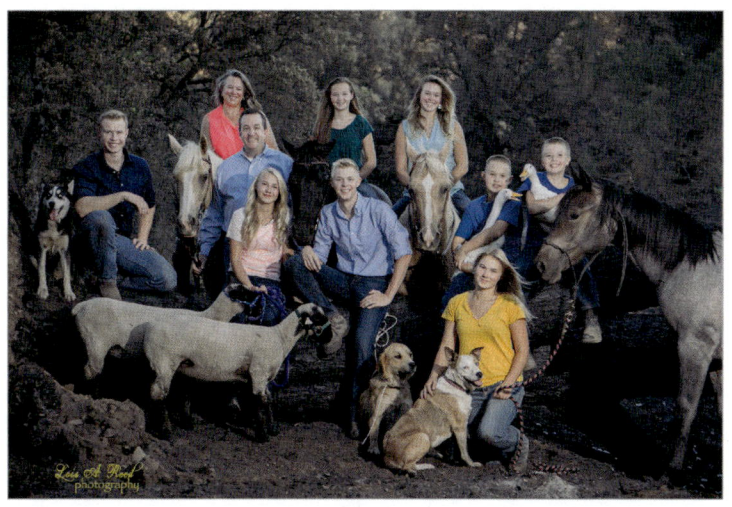

Our family on our ranch in Mariposa with some of our animals. I am on the left with my Mom, and sisters Margaret and Katie on the horses. In front of them are my father, Bernadette, Bernhard, and my two little brothers, William and Karl. Analise is in the front. Sadly, my older brother, Matthew is missing. He had just gotten married and was living in another state.

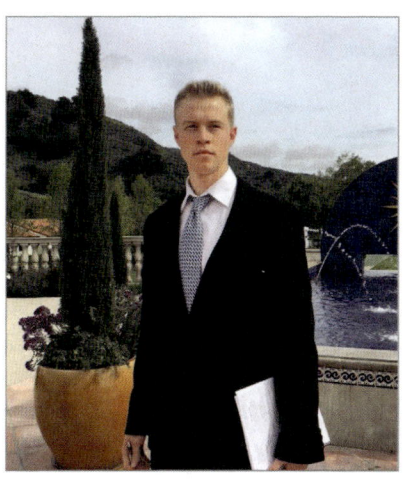

Right before my thesis defense at Thomas Aquinas College.

CHAPTER 2

DENTAL PREP

U nfortunately, due to the liberal arts nature of the college, I was not able to fulfill all of my prerequisites for dental school. I needed to take an additional two years at local universities to fulfill the necessary requirements. I buckled down and got ready for two more years of school before finally beginning my dream. I was thrilled when a local dental office took a chance on me and hired me to be a dental assistant. I was very excited to begin work, and knew it would give me an edge over my future classmates. It would help me explore the world of dentistry and open my eyes to the bigger picture before I committed to it.

I took my first prerequisite courses at Fresno State which was an hour and a half away. I needed to make this drive three days a week; however, the long drive offered me plenty of time to contemplate life, my future, and my priorities. I made a point of spending at least five to ten minutes of the drive in silence. This time was always precious to me, taking a moment to step out of the busywork and get away from distractions. I was able to center myself on what was most important, namely, my faith and my responsibilities to God. It was in these moments that I would reflect on what God's will was for me. A prayer that I kept making in my heart was asking our Lord to give me direction and to tell me if I was doing the right thing. I felt consolation in knowing that if I just kept making the most of the opportunities in my life and leaving the direction to him, he would not let me go astray. I often recited in my head the lines from Psalm 23 knowing that he would guide my path in this life:

> The Lord is my shepherd; I shall not want. He makes me lie down in green pastures; he leads me beside still waters; he restores my soul. He leads me in right paths for his name's sake. Even though I walk through the darkest valley, I fear no evil; for you are with me; your rod and your staff they comfort me. (Psalm 23:1–4)

I would encourage each and every one of you who are reading this to take the time daily to find a moment of silence to listen and pray to God. It might be in the morning, or in the evening, or a brief pause in the middle of the day. But either way, take the opportunity to ask our Lord what his will is for you, and ask him to guide your thoughts and your desires, so that you may follow the path that he has for you. I am constantly amazed at how these little moments have played such a profound role in my life, often helping me feel more confident about a decision, or look at things from another perspective. Allow our Lord to intervene and the Holy Spirit to guide your decisions in life. It is important that we earnestly seek God's help and his will for us and not obstinately hold on to our own. May we always find time each day to look at God, thank him for all that he has given us, and ask that he might help us to be his instruments in the world.

Despite the long commute, and the long hours, I did very well at Fresno State, knocking out one more year of prerequisites before dental school. I enjoyed my routine of going to school, rollerblading across the long pathways and parking lots to get to class, bouncing between my study group and the library, blowing things up in the lab, taking naps in my car, and going out to eat with my friends after a long day.

When it came time for my final year of prerequisites, I found that the University of California, Merced, which was closer by about forty-five minutes, had exactly the class I needed. However, when I applied, I was told that all priority went to the full-time students. There was no guarantee I could take the class and there was nothing I could do to increase my chances. I didn't know what to do. If I didn't get into this class, I would have to wait an additional year to get into dental school. Trying not to feel defeated, I prayed that no one was interested in taking high-level science classes, or at least not enough people to fill the class up. On the first day of school, I went to the office to see if there was any room for me. They told me that I had to wait a week to allow students to change or add a class. Furthermore, they told me I had to pay for all my classes before I even knew if I had gotten in. I was stunned. I had to call home to borrow money from everyone because I didn't have enough in my bank account. I was told I would be reimbursed if I couldn't get into class, but it was small consolation and I was very stressed. To add insult to injury, they told me I had to figure out what books were used in the class, buy the books and study them while waiting so I didn't fall behind. They wouldn't even let me access the online portal, so I couldn't even turn in assignments. I had to accept that I would just be docked points for anything I missed during the first week.

It was nerve-racking to say the least, knowing that classes had already started, I had no access to any of the information, and was not even sure if I had a spot for a whole week. I talked to the teacher outside of class, and he thankfully allowed me to follow along by giving me the the reading assignments. I studied as if I was in the class and hoped. We all rejoiced when I finally got the notification that I was in. Thankfully, I was not too far behind, and any of the assignments I missed were small enough that they wouldn't affect my grade significantly. It was a rough start, but I buckled down and started my last year of prerequisites.

While taking classes at UC Merced, I continued to work as a dental assistant in Mariposa. I enjoyed the work immensely and learned so much from everybody there, discussing business, dental techniques, and cutting-edge software used in the dental field. My work hours seemed to fly by as I was surrounded by friends and future colleagues. This was, for sure, one thing I was going to miss when I had to leave and go to dental school.

Halfway through the year, I started working on my application. I compiled all of my transcripts and filled out the general questionnaire. Then came time for my last two things: letters of recommendation and the Dental Aptitude Test, the latter being the biggest challenge for me in getting into dental school. I sent out letters to my teachers and the dentist that I was working for. All that was left was to work hard studying for the DAT.

Every day after school I committed myself to studying for the DAT. First, I went to adoration at a nearby church, prayed for fifteen minutes, and then to a nearby coffee shop, ordered a large iced coffee and went to work. Four or five hours went by before my head started hurting and I couldn't read any more words on the page. I finished up my study session by grabbing a quick dinner nearby and headed home. These study sessions were crucial to my preparation for the DAT, and helped prepare me for the long hours of studying that were to come in dental school.

The most difficult sections of the test involved classes that I'd never taken, and so I had to teach myself from scratch. Despite the challenge, I knew if I put in the hard work studying, I would be able to achieve the results I wanted. I continued my study routine for the next three months—dental assisting on my off days, and going to school, adoration, and the coffee shop on the other days. My body and mind fell into a rhythm. I felt good about the progress I was making and decided to schedule my test date for the following month.

It was finally the day of the test. After so many days of preparation, I felt ready, but I knew it wasn't going to be easy. It was five hours long, and it seemed equally possible that I could pass or fail. I stepped into the room, said a prayer, and started the test. The hours seemed to drag by as my brain gradually became more and more cloudy from reading so much text on the small screen and taxing my brain by pulling from the deepest recesses of my mind. I was allowed a small break in the middle, where I got to eat a granola bar, drink some water, and gather my thoughts. The small break gave me the stamina to finish the second half. I went back determined, hyped myself up, and started flying through the second section. By the time I got to the end, I was exhausted. I wanted nothing more than to walk out of that room but I made sure to use all of my time wisely and go back over any questions that I was uncertain about before finally clicking SUBMIT.

Unlike most exams, where you have to wait several weeks or even months before getting your results, the DAT results were instant, and I knew as soon as I clicked that button I would see whether or not I had done enough to get into dental school. I said another prayer as my heart was pounding through my chest, closed my eyes, and pushed the button. I half opened my eyes and prayed that I would see a good result. The screen gradually processed and gave me my final score.

I crushed it! Not only did I pass, but I did exceptionally well. I could feel the heavy weight lift off my shoulders. I was so thankful that all my hard work had paid off, and I knew that I would be able to get into dental school. My future career started piecing itself together in my head. With the final barrier removed, now I was ready to start dental school. It felt like the beginning of the rest of my life. I thanked God once again, giving all glory to him, and picked up the phone to call my parents and tell them the good news. They congratulated me and got excited, joining in to discuss where I should apply, and what that decision would mean for my future.

I talked to a lot of people and checked a lot of sources to determine what was the best dental school. Despite a lot of good reasons for the other schools, I knew the school that I most wanted to get into was University of the Pacific, UOP. They were known for producing some of the best technical dentists in the country and were renowned for the expertise and leadership of their students upon graduating. It was a three-year accelerated program, and I knew if I got the military scholarship that would mean saving two years of my life, because I would only have to pay back three years of service after graduating instead of the traditional four.

The terms of the scholarship were one year of service for every year of school.

Not only that, but the school was located in San Francisco, which was only a three-hour drive from home. This would make it much easier to visit my family more often. After taking the DAT, and receiving my letters of recommendation, I was finally ready to submit my application.

I knew that the school was highly competitive, so I made sure to visit before I turned in my application and get some face time with the admissions committee and any of the teachers there. I enjoyed visiting and loved the atmosphere. The school motto was "at UOP we make leaders, and along the way they become dentists." The idea of focusing on building people up to be the best they could be and focusing so heavily on leadership and humanity was very appealing to me. I knew how integral that mindset was to both business and life. That was one of the reasons I went to a liberal arts college, and made it even more clear that this was the school for me. After talking to several of the students and hearing the same thing, I realized I was in good company. It was clear that my colleagues would also be interested in pursuing knowledge and dentistry in the same way that I was. After leaving the campus, I didn't even have to think twice. This was the only school I wanted to attend. A couple of weeks later I pressed SUBMIT on my application, said a prayer, and hoped for the best.

After getting my application turned in, I was far from done. It was not until I got accepted that I would hear back about the military scholarship, but I kept talking to the recruiter, made sure all of my ducks were in a row, and tried to determine the likelihood that I would be able to get the scholarship, as my future greatly depended on it.

Like most good things in life, I had to be patient and wait to hear back. However, I did not let my time slip away, making the most of it by studying dentistry, and working hard to learn as much as I could from podcasts, dental assisting, and books. I couldn't wait to get started. I had always loved working with my hands and loved woodcarving. Many afternoons, I sat outside our home and carved animals out of blocks of wood with a rotary tool. As I worked with the wood, I imagined what it would be like to practice dentistry. The idea of helping get rid of disease and rebuilding a smile into something beautiful was always in the back of my mind, and I knew that it would be a big part of my life.

During this time, I pushed myself both mentally and physically in the gym, working out and staying fit. I loved going to the gym after a long day of work and working out. It felt good to push myself to the point of exertion and then just a little bit further. I made many friendships, formed by the common goal of being fit and strong. The culmination of my physical accomplishments was competing in multiple Spartan races across California. For those not familiar with the Spartan race, it is an obstacle course mixed in with a run ranging from three to thirteen miles. There are three difficulties of the Spartan race: The first is a Spartan Sprint, which is approximately three miles with twenty obstacles, the second is a Spartan Super, which is approximately six miles with twenty-five obstacles, and the third is a Spartan Beast with approximately thirteen miles and thirty obstacles. The culmination of my challenge came when I completed the trifecta, finishing all three, and a bonus on top was placing in the top 4 percent of my age group during the Spartan Sprint.

But always in the back of my mind was my application to UOP. Months went by as I waited, and there was still no word. I calmed my excited nerves, reminding myself that I didn't expect to hear back until September when they started calling out for interviews. When September finally hit, I reached out to some of my friends who I knew had also applied to see if they'd heard anything. Most of them were still waiting, but one of them said that he got an interview, and immediately, my brain began to panic. I knew it was a competitive school, and I had applied to only one school. This was by far the best school, according to all of my research, and this made the decision concrete. I knew that even if I didn't get in this year, it was still worth it to apply again next year. But the thought of putting off dental school for a whole year left me anxious. I was ready to start at UOP and begin my life as a dentist. I kept saying novenas and praying that I would hear good news soon.

Work and school continued as normal until one day at the gym, while I was running on the treadmill, I got a call. I glanced down, and between my heavy breathing and the pounding of the background music, saw that it was a call from San Francisco. I immediately pulled the plug on the treadmill and tried to catch my breath before picking up. I put the phone to my sweaty ear and tried to answer calmly. It was a call from the admissions office at the University of Pacific dental school. Somehow my heart was beating even faster than when I was on the treadmill. I waited with bated breath as the admissions coordinator got straight to the point and told me that I'd been selected for an interview and would like to schedule a day for me to come in. A sigh of relief managed to sneak in between my heavy breathing, and I calmly selected a day that would work, trying my best not to burst out excitedly at the good news. I thanked him before hanging up. I immediately said an internal prayer of thanksgiving before calling my parents to let them know the good news.

Celebration and partying, acknowledging one more step in the process that I'd spent the last ten years working toward. But I was not out of the woods yet, I still needed to have the interview and get accepted. I started preparing for interview questions—going through my résumé and my application, finding any weaknesses and having an explanation for them, trying to figure out what strengths I had and how to highlight them, learning more about the dental school and any trivia that I could squeeze in to make myself look like a better fit. There were so many suggestions and strategies tossed around by my siblings. Trying my best to prepare without really knowing what to prepare for.

When the day finally came, I felt well rested and excited, although a bit nervous. I dressed nicely in a suit with a matching blue tie, hopped in the car and drove across the bay into San Francisco. I had visited the school once before, so thankfully I knew where to park and how to navigate the streets. I walked in once again, my heart pounding, and greeted everyone nicely. I explained that I was there for an interview. They gave me a name tag and let me know that it would just be a moment, so I should make myself comfortable. I hung out and chatted with a couple of other applicants who were also there for interviews. I tried to size up the competition and see where I ranked in terms of grades and the DAT, constantly assessing the likelihood of being accepted from among my peers. There were a lot of strong applicants, but I felt like I was among them and had a fair shot.

The interviewers gathered us over and told us they were ready to begin the interviews. They assured us that this was a very relaxed and laid-back interview process, because they were just trying to get to know us, not grill us for answers.

I imagined that they wanted to see a positive attitude and evaluate whether we would make a good match with the school. My first interview was with a teacher who had been teaching for many years at UOP. She asked me questions about my life, a couple of questions about my résumé, and then just had a general conversation with me about why I was interested in dentistry and what excited me about the school and my future. The conversation was very relaxing, and I felt like I was compelling, simply because I really loved the career, and I was passionate about helping people and making a difference in the dental world. Judging by her body language, I felt pretty good when we shook hands, and I moved on to the next step.

In the next part of the interviews, they had us meet with a faculty member. Once again it was a very relaxing conversation about futures, careers, family, life, and morals. It felt so good to just talk and get to know these amazing people. With every conversation, I was more and more reassured that this was the right choice, and these were the people that I wanted to work with. I felt good as we finished the interview and finally moved onto the last part where we met with the students so that we could see once again how our relationship was on the peer-to-peer level. We met in the simulation lab, where many hours of hard work and practice took place, learning dental techniques on manikins. Curious, I asked several questions about the layout of the school and the difficulty. They replied honestly saying that it was very intense, very difficult, but if you managed your time well, you would learn a lot. They also told me that the instructors were very good, and although harsh, it just made you a better dentist and improved your skills to a level more capable than any other school in the US. I asked some follow-up questions about different parts of the coursework, the surrounding area and housing. But all of the conversation seemed to flow together nicely, and I was already excited to be part of this family. I hoped that my application would be accepted so that I could join them in the fall. They gave us a couple more presentations about finances, tuition options, and financial aid, and briefly went over military scholarships. It was very helpful information, information that I knew would make a big difference for many other people. However, since I'd already made up my mind, it was just extra information so that I could plan accordingly for the future. The day came to a close, and I said goodbye to everyone, headed to the car and drove home. I prayed a rosary on the way home asking God to help direct my process and open up an application spot for me to attend next year. I got home and told everyone the good news. I told them that it was a very successful interview, and that I was hoping to hear back in the next month or so.

In the meantime, I followed up with the military scholarship. I made the call to my recruiter and asked about the next steps. He gave me a couple of preliminary forms to fill out but said the big-ticket item was getting accepted to dental school. Other than that, I had everything turned in, and just had to wait till I heard back from the school. There was a sigh of relief, and a slight gulp of worry, as I realized that so much rested on the decision of the school. My family and I started another novena for the success of my application and we waited patiently to hear back.

Waiting for something builds patience, and more importantly, shows us the reality of depending on someone else to get what we want. Patience is very close to humility, and waiting is an act of submission, submitting to the constraints of time and the power outside of ourselves. Patience helps combat pride and gives us a chance to reflect upon the fact that we are not the center of the universe. There is a power that is far greater than ourselves. We must give ourselves to God and always place him as a priority in our life. Sometimes God makes this easier for us by giving us crosses to direct our attention back to him. Unfortunately, we have found so many ways to block out God's subtle pointers that we can often fail to see his influence in our lives. The next time that you are required to wait for something, and are struggling to have the patience for it, remember to submit your will to God, to recognize his power and greatness above your own, and let his timing be what guides you, so that all things might bring us closer to him.

Just like so many other times in my life, I got home one day after school to see my family anxiously gathered around the table, where a letter sat alone on the table. I could see immediately that it was from the University of Pacific dental school. My heart was beating at a thousand miles a minute, and I knew that so much hard work culminated in this one moment in time. It felt like my entire future was in my hands, and it would all come down to the next several seconds. I didn't hesitate. I immediately opened the letter and read the first lines. Congratulations! You have been accepted…I didn't even finish reading it, I knew that my dreams had come true, and I would be attending dental school in the fall.

Once again, we celebrated. Everything felt right. All of my hard work was finally starting to pay off, and there was a light at the end of the tunnel. All those long hours driving to school, all of the stress of trying to find the classes I needed, all of the money, time, and commitment that I had put into learning this profession. I was ready. I knew this was only the beginning, but it was another crucial step in what I imagined would be the rest of my life.

Good news following upon good news, I also found out that I was awarded a full-ride military scholarship into the US Navy. Not only was I going to my dream school, but I also wasn't going to come out with any debt. The deal was that I would serve for three years after graduating in exchange for my full tuition and a monthly stipend. It was a scary thought, to sign a contract binding my life and my career to the military so far in the future, but I was confident it was the right step, and I was excited to serve our country and be debt free.

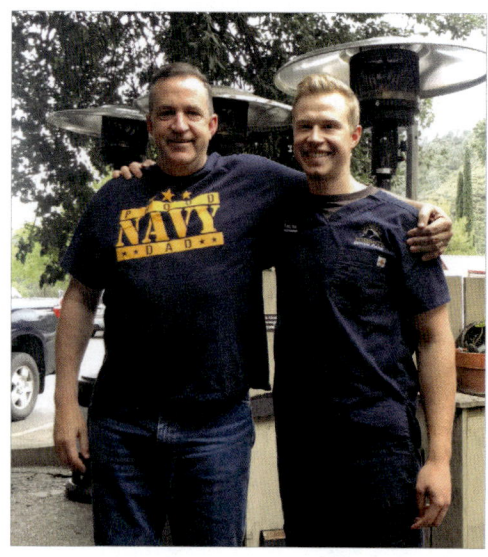

My father was very proud that I had joined the Navy and made sure to "buy the T-shirt."

Pushing Through the Pain

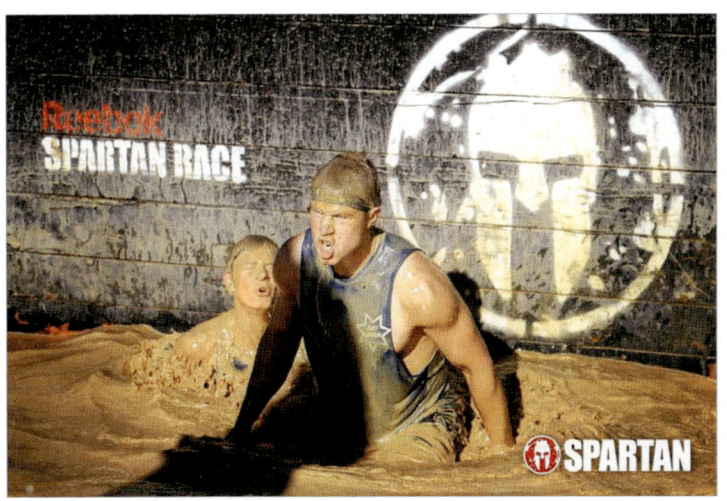

My brother, Bernhard, and I competing in a Spartan Race.

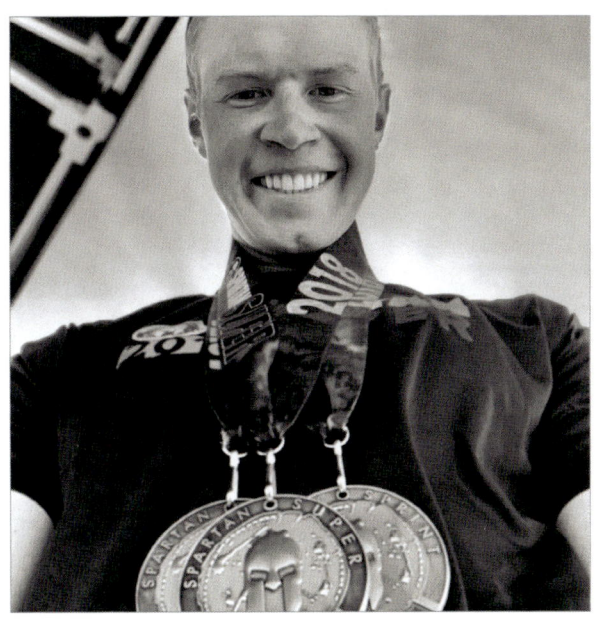

My three medals after I had won the Trifecta

CHAPTER 3

UNIVERSITY OF THE PACIFIC

The time finally came for me to go to dental school. This was a big one. I was going to be living on my own, not in a dorm, but in a house, where I would have to figure out how to provide myself with all the basic necessities. It would mean figuring out where the gym was, figuring out where a local laundromat was, figuring out when street cleaning was, and figuring out where I could go grocery shopping. It would be a lot easier if it wasn't in San Francisco, where everything was so much more chaotic and stressful. Not to mention the high crime rate, and vast homeless population. I knew I would have to keep my head on a swivel and plan ahead for safety and parking. I had my family help me move in and buy furniture to renovate my new place so that it was ready to go. I decided to live the first three months with a fellow schoolmate of mine to allow me to get my bearings before finding my own place.

When dental school began, I was nervous. I was suddenly afraid that it would not be what I had dreamed of all these years. However, as soon as my classes began and I started to get to work, my fear dissipated. All of my unique skills and capabilities fit perfectly in the dental environment, and I was enjoying every second of it. Even the late nights studying I enjoyed, knowing that I was building my expertise for a lifelong profession.

Despite the difficult coursework, I sought out every opportunity to expand my horizons and take on new challenges. I joined several clubs and volunteered as the CDA (California Dental Association) student delegate for our class. The extra work was fulfilling, and I was happy to provide my insights and any information I could to improve the school programs. I enjoyed networking and interacting with my peers and with dentists that had already graduated.

Everything was going great, and I was enjoying my new responsibilities, when out of nowhere, Covid hit. Everything went into lockdown, and we were all sent home. There were several weeks of confusion as the school tried to figure out how to make up for lost time and how to make everything virtual. They gave us homework, told us to keep studying, and said they would instruct us on the new format for virtual learning. It was difficult at first, but I was quickly able to figure out how to succeed and what study plan I needed to use. The only thing that was missing from our virtual learning experience was the clinic. It was hard learning to be a dentist without actually being able to see patients. The school front-loaded our semester with coursework education, opting to postpone the clinic until they could figure it out. A couple of months went by, and they finally told us that everything would be postponed till the start of the next year. At this point, no one knew what was going on or how long Covid would last, but they had high hopes for returning next year in full force. We buckled down on our learning and passed our classes as we waited out the storm and waited to hear back about the next year.

That spring and summer, I got to spend a lot of time with my family. All my brothers and sisters had also been sent home, and many had brought along friends who didn't want to be stuck in the city with nowhere to go. The house was full of people, conversations, and lots of multitasking. One morning, all of us were cooking breakfast while holding our laptops and doing Zoom classes. Of course, we were on mute with our photo avatar up so the classroom couldn't see the gourmet breakfast unfolding. Even though everything was still in lockdown, having a forty-acre farm definitely allowed for many ways to enjoy our time together. We swam in our stream, had outdoor barbecues, rode horses, and built our own zip lines. My parents happily gave us projects to do on the farm, and in the cool of the afternoon we played football and Ultimate Frisbee. In the evenings, we enjoyed heated arguments about the politics behind Covid, and what the future would look like. Because the world was on lockdown, everyone got to enjoy more time together, whether it was working from home or just being home from school. So, while it might not have been ideal, we still were able to make the most of it and had a really great time together.

The first year of school passed by in the blink of an eye, and I found myself at the top of the class. All of the nights of late hours studying, all of the work that I put into prerequisites, all of the work that I had done practicing my hand skills through wood carving, and finally all of my work as a dental assistant, were now coming to fruition. We were finally done with practicing on manikins and would be starting in the clinic working on real people. I was excited about the new year and to start seeing patients. I knew this was a big step and that I would now be able to make good use of my talents to help people.

Year two started, and Covid was still in full force, but thankfully, the city gave us special permission to start treating patients again, albeit with extreme precaution. We immediately got back to work. At first, the instruments felt a little awkward in my hands, but after a short time I got back into the swing of things and the instruments quickly felt like an extension of my hands. My group-practice leader, who knew my skill, gave me a special assignment to see a patient earlier than other students because she needed an emergency procedure. I jumped on board excitedly, not quite knowing what I was signing myself up for.

After all the paperwork was done, I went in for my first examination. The patient was going on a trip and her tooth was causing her pain. I put on my special dental magnifying glasses, called loupes, and took a look. She was missing half of her tooth on one of her back molars. I determined that I had to do a temporary crown to help hold the tooth together before she went on her trip. Looking at a real patient in the chair, waiting for me and trusting me, I was nervous. My heart raced and my blood was pumping fast. I took a deep breath and calmed myself down. It did not help that with all of the additional Covid regulations, I was trying to breathe through three masks, a face shield, and loupes. Needless to say, everything got fogged up within the first ten seconds. I slowed my breathing and focused on my task. I cleaned my mask every thirty seconds and took my time so that I could do the best I knew how. I had help from a senior who walked me through the whole process and helped calm my nerves. Thankfully, at that point, all of my movements felt like instinct, and I was able to get the job done.

When I finally looked down after checking the bite and polishing the tooth, I couldn't believe what I had just made. This was my first patient and it was such a big filling. I had done a good job and I was extremely proud of myself. The patient was happy and went their way, and life went on. I will always remember that patient, and how nervous I was to do my first filling. It was stressful and terrifying, but in the end so rewarding to be able to see that my work could bring someone out of pain and provide them with the new opportunity to chew and smile. What a great feeling it was! After the first patient, I got several more, and quickly booked out my schedule for the next month. This was the culmination of all of those years of working so hard. All my skill and expertise were helping people, and I could finally feel the rewards of a job well-done.

How could I have ever guessed that I was dancing on a cliff, and my entire life was about to crumble before me. It was only a couple of months later that a buddy of mine, my old roommate, asked me to join him on a weeklong ski trip over Thanksgiving break. I agreed happily, always being fond of adventure, never realizing how that ski trip would change the course of my life forever.

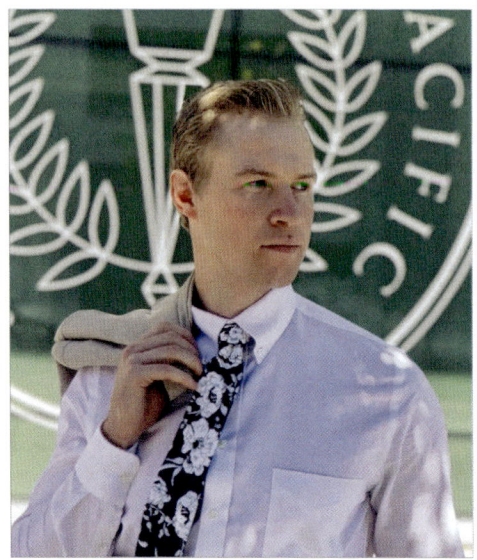
Photo outside University of the Pacific.

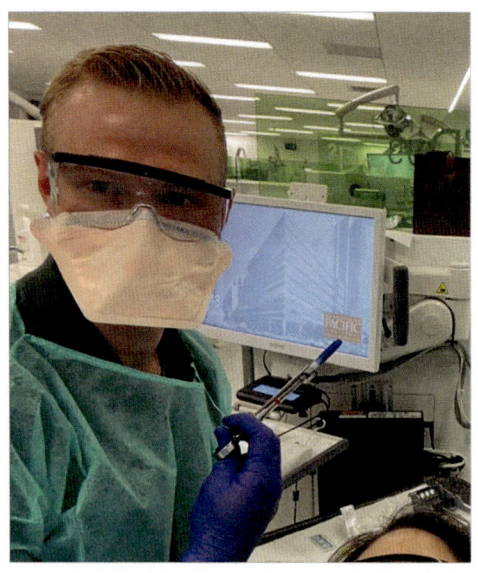
Working on my first patient at UOP.

CHAPTER 4

INTO THE BEYOND

The plan was simple: we would have a week off for Thanksgiving break, and because I was part of the military, I got a season pass for next to nothing. We planned on going out to Tahoe for a week and trying several ski resorts. To save money, we packed the back of the car with a mattress and blankets so we could just car camp wherever we went. We left early in the morning and got to Tahoe in time to prepare everything and make sure all of our lift tickets and gear were ready to go for the following morning. We started off in southern Tahoe skiing at Heavenly Valley and enjoyed several days skiing down the mountain and taking in the sights. After a couple of days we decided to check out another resort and settled on NorthStar. We headed out in the evening so that we would be good to go the next morning. Once we got there, we checked that everything was good, got some food, and settled in for the night so that we could get an early start on the next day. I sent a photo to my family that night. Our grins covered our faces from ear to ear! I had missed Thanksgiving at home but we were having the time of our lives!

We awoke to frost-covered windows, and as we cracked the seal on the car door, letting an icy breeze in, a burst of adrenaline shot through us, and we couldn't wait to get out on the new slopes. We grabbed a coffee and headed out. We got to the resort just after sunrise and hopped in line for the ski gondola, enjoying the fresh mountain air and the beautiful views. As we rode to the top, we caught sight of some of the ski slopes to our left and right. The snow looked pretty good, although a little icy because it was still early in the season. Our hopes and spirits were high, and after a couple of small runs on the lower mountain to get ourselves warmed up, we took the ski lift all the way to the top and started going down some much harder black diamond slopes. Everything was feeling great, and we were enjoying the nice weather and the challenging runs.

After a couple more runs, we took a snack break. I mentioned to my friend that I was interested in trying a ski jump, since this resort was known for its well-developed terrain parks. I had seen the terrain park coming up the gondola and knew that it was marked as a family friendly zone on the ski map, so I figured it was something I could try without having to worry too much about the danger. We discussed it a little more, then he told me that if I wanted to hit a jump, I had to make sure to full-send it, so that I didn't chicken out halfway up and hurt myself. I nodded in agreement and then we headed back out.

As we were coming off the top of the mountain, we hit some smaller slopes on the way down and made our way over toward the terrain park. We slowed down as we came into it, and I quickly tried out the balance beam. I was surprised at how slippery it was, and immediately slid off; however, my courage was not daunted and I got back up, ready to try out the jump. My friend's words from earlier echoed in my head. "If you're gonna take a jump, you've just got to full send it." Adrenaline was pumping through my veins, and I was ready to go. I tucked my poles and took off down the remaining fifty yards of the terrain park toward the jump.

There were two smaller jumps on either end with one big jump in the center. I went back and forth in my head about which one I would do. However, in the end I decided that if I was going to do a jump, I might as well do it right and headed straight for the big one. I started gaining a lot of speed and steadied my body for the jump. Air flying past my face. Ready to free myself from earth and gravity. Into the beyond.

I anticipated the movements I needed to guide my body safely over the jump. Suddenly something was wrong. My mind struggled to figure out what was different. The shadows from the trees distorted the landscape. I didn't see that the ground dipped before the jump. I found out later this was intentional, to give the skiers a bigger jump. But the hollow in the snow was not clearly marked, and I didn't expect it. All I knew was that out of nowhere the ground had given way beneath my feet. The sudden change threw me backwards and I flew off the jump feet first. As soon as I was in the air, I knew I was in for a bad landing. I didn't panic, I remained calm, relaxed, and thought that maybe I could just bounce my way out of this.

However, bouncing back was not in store for me that day. Instead, I hit the icy snow with a resounding smack as both my hips and tailbone landed first on the snow and immediately blew out of their sockets. The remaining force whiplashed through my neck and snapped my C6 vertebrae. I lay there motionless, fully conscious, taking in my surroundings and my situation. I knew immediately I was paralyzed, my whole body felt warm, and I couldn't distinguish any of my limbs.

    I was in shock and felt oddly calm. I did not scream or cry out. I felt disconnected from my body as though I was watching from outside myself. I assured myself that "my body" was close enough to get help. My friend saw my crash and I knew that all the necessary medical attention would be coming my way shortly. I lay there, waiting as I heard the information in the background regarding transportation. I listened with an odd detachment as they tried to decide between an ambulance and a helicopter, and after some debate, they settled on the helicopter. I heard an ETA of five minutes.

    I closed my eyes as I felt the wind sting my face and heard the sound of the helicopter blades cutting through the frigid air. Next thing I knew, I was being lifted up into the air and transported to the hospital. It was at this point that I started to pass out, letting exhaustion and shock take me.

    I woke up to find that I was being carted into a surgery room and getting a phone call from my mother, asking me, "Do you know what is happening?" "

    I was calm and answered her, "Yes, I do. I am paralyzed and they will be doing surgery to help stabilize my spine."

    She paused for a moment and then said, "All that has happened is by God's will and for the salvation of souls."

    I was filled with conviction and responded, "That is the most important thing."

    She seemed consoled to hear this and managed to squeeze out one final I love you before I had to go. I told her I loved her too and then I went into surgery. That was the last time I was able to speak for almost fifty days.

The next forty days that followed were a blur, but what I do remember scares me even to this day. Just recalling some of the images and situations that I went through fills me with such great fear and dread that I can barely breathe. Panic sets in and causes me to nearly shake with the horror of it all. However, I think it is important to write what I can remember, so I will find the courage to recall them and recount what I can.

My earliest memories are less images, and more sensations and feelings. I remember being slowly choked by a feeding tube going down the back of my throat through my nose and then a bigger tube also going down my throat, and because of this I could not speak. I remember the terror of not being able to call out if I needed help. I was completely at the mercy of the nurses around me. I felt trapped inside my body, and unable to escape, forced to witness all of the horrors to come without any way to block them out. It was a living hell. Despite my arms not being fully paralyzed, they were so weak that I did not have the strength to push a call button, and so there was no way I could signal the nurses. What I didn't realize was that my arms were tied down because I was so insistent on pulling out the tubes that kept me alive. My mind knew that all of these things were foreign and not natural and I didn't want them and had no perspective that I needed them.

When my mother was finally allowed to see me, she was horrified. I had a ventilator down my throat into my lungs to bring oxygen to them. I had a c-spine brace protecting my neck. Because my hips were blown out, I had clamps screwed into my bones on each side of each leg slowly pulling my legs back into place. I had multiple wires monitoring my oxygen, my breathing, and my pulse. I was under massive drugs so as to stay just awake to live but not alert enough to fight. Even under so many drugs, I bit through a few of the ventilator tubes and struggled against my restraints. My mother said I looked like a trapped lion. But I felt much weaker and more defeated than that.

I thought to myself, this is where I die, surrounded by nurses and doctors, unable to call out or ask for help. In that time of darkness, I called out to our Lord, asking for the strength of perseverance, and offering it up for the salvation of the world. Lines from Psalm 143 echoed through my mind like both a prayer and a taunt:

> I am crushed to the ground;
> he makes me dwell in the darkness
> like those long dead.
> So my spirit grows faint within me;
> my heart within me is dismayed.
> I remember the days of long ago;
> I meditate on all your works
> and consider what your hands have done.
> I spread out my hands to you;
> I thirst for you like a parched land.
> Answer me quickly, Lord; my spirit fails.

The hospital room was dark, and since it was wintertime, my windows faced the west and never caught the sun. The shades seemed always drawn. As my memory faded in and out because of the drugs I was on, I struggled to live. One such moment was when I got very bad pneumonia, and they had to suction out my lungs by shoving a tube down my throat and pumping my lungs full of saline. It was painful and the process seemed to go on for an eternity. After that a volcano of mucus erupted out of my mouth. I panicked, feeling the mucus covering my nostrils and mouth. I was worried that I wouldn't be able to breathe. I didn't understand that I was breathing through the ventilator. My mind didn't have the ability to put that together, and the experience seemed very similar to how people describe waterboarding, where even though they are not drowning, the mind convinces them that they are.

Finally, the doctors determined I was well enough to take out the ventilator and put in a tracheotomy. The tube was out of my throat! There was the promise of putting in a speaking valve, but still my lungs were not strong enough for that. It was now possible to reduce some of the drugs in my system, allowing me to be more conscious. This was a blessing, but also allowed me a greater awareness of my situation. I battled severe depression, and had terrible nightmares, torturing me. I looked forward to my mom's visits. She told me stories of home, which sometimes made me sad. She showed me the video of my dog, Nova, and her new puppies. She read to me my favorite book, *The Perfect Joy of St. Francis*, and prayed countless rosaries with only my mind to join her since I could not speak. And many times, she just sat with me in silence, trying to absorb my pain. The greatest blessing was when she brought me a very holy priest who brought me the sacraments and prayed a rosary with me. These were the only things that kept me going in a sea of darkness and despair.

When I first started physical therapy, they tried to get me to sit up. It was terrifying to see how exhausting it was. In fact, the first time they managed to sit me up, I passed out, my heart stopped, and I coded. My mom was in the hospital hall and heard the death code and what was going on in my room over the speaker. After the doctors revived me, she rushed to me sobbing. She wouldn't stop crying and I tried to tell her it would be okay. It broke my heart to hear her cry like that. She finally gathered herself and asked me what it was like. She made a little joke and asked if I had seen a bright light. Then she laughed and said, "Don't go near the bright light." I smiled. But I didn't dare tell her how easy it felt to just stop breathing and stop struggling. Maybe there was no bright light, but there was a sweet break from the hell I was living in. In fact, I coded five more times over the following weeks, battling right on the edge of life and death.

There were a few moments that brought me genuine joy during my stay, among them were the amazing nurses and care team that I had. I remember them all being like beautiful angels, helping me and being there for me.

Eventually, I worked up enough strength to be able to sit up for about thirty minutes, and so they offered me a trip outside in my hospital bed, thinking that my blood pressure was stable enough to handle the brief trip. Even though it wasn't a lot, I was excited to go outside. It had been forever since I'd seen anything except the walls of my hospital room. As we made our way down the hallway, my mind wandered toward the golden afternoons back home in Mariposa. The warm sun beating down on my face, the birds in the background, and the gentle breeze.

When I finally got to the door, it opened with a giant whoosh, and what I imagined could not have been further from the truth. There was no sun, the temperature was thirty degrees, and all I could see was concrete and building windows. My one journey outside was the final straw, and internally I broke down. I was depressed and struggling with the ability to continue. I wanted my life to be over, and not have to deal with it anymore.

For forty days and forty nights I battled death over and over again in the ICU. I did not realize that my father was in a hotel room attached to the hospital, praying for me. It must have broken his heart to be so near to me, but not able to visit. I did not realize that there was a miraculous surge of prayers flooding over my soul: friends, strangers, classrooms of children, monasteries and convents all praying for my recovery. My mom wrote of my journey in such a compelling way that strangers texted my parents telling them they were coming back to the faith. It was a strange and grace-filled time, but I was not aware. I battled death and despair alone in my dark and sunless room.

Two of the saddest days were Christmas and my brother's wedding. Christmas has always been a special holiday for me, and my favorite part was to think very carefully about what people wanted for Christmas, and then buy it for them and watch their faces light up as they opened it.

However, this Christmas was horrible. My mother wanted to stay at the hospital with me, but not only were there eight children who wanted their mother home for Christmas, but my brother was getting married soon after. And so even though it broke my heart in a thousand ways, I told her she must go home. When she left, I felt as though I was left for dead in a dark grave. I was stuck in the bed, half alive, while the nurses struggled to put on a TV stream of Christmas Mass. While waiting for them to figure out which channel it was on, there was a holiday cartoon show about how different cultures celebrated Christmas. While I'm sure the show was decent, that day, it was straight out of a nightmare, it was terrifying, and strange. Nothing that I knew of Christmas was being portrayed, and I felt even more alone. And despite tons of presents, and even more Christmas cards, I felt trapped, buried, and dead inside. This was the closest to being buried alive that I could imagine.

The second day that broke my heart was my brother's wedding. A couple of months before my accident, he had asked me to be his best man. A request that still means the world to me. I was so incredibly honored to be asked and couldn't wait to help him celebrate his wedding.

Days before the accident, I began preparing a best man speech that I would never deliver. Jokes, laughs, and more importantly, the excellences of his character that I would never be able to tell the world. On the day of his wedding; the nurses were very sweet. They figured out a way that they could livestream me at the reception so that everyone could see. They got a shirt, a tie, a big sign that said "Congratulations" and some balloons. They planned to put a speaking valve on the trach, and we hoped I would be strong enough to say a few words to the happy couple on their wedding day.

It pains me to go back in time and remember what it was like, the sorrow and sadness of not being there and not being able to celebrate with them. The anguish of not being able to dance and party and live that moment with them. When it was time to speak, I forced myself, as much as I could, to concentrate and build up the strength just to mumble a few words. My mind was foggy from all of the drugs, and my body was weak, since I was still dependent on the trach to give me oxygen. Every word felt like it would suffocate me. I finally drew the strength to impart the most important words that I could think of: "Stay close to Mary and our heavenly father. Your faith is the most important thing in this life. Do not take it for granted and always pray for the strength to hold onto that faith. May God bless you both, goodbye."

The simple few sentences were enough to almost make me pass out from exhaustion, and waves of sadness washed over me as they disconnected the line on the livestream. I'll never forget seeing the faces of so many people that I love, knowing that I was missing out on this occasion and would never get to experience it again. At the wedding everyone was crying, including my brother Bernhard and his new bride. He tried to joke saying, "Thanks Franz, for making everyone cry at my wedding." But the laughter could not pierce the overwhelming grief of separation and loss.

I felt sorry for myself, but I also felt sorry for my family and friends who had to live through this moment with their hearts being touched both by joy, and by sadness. I wanted to disappear. My heart was so broken, my spirit so low. All in one instant, everything I had always wanted and would never have was playing out before my eyes. All I remember is just continually praying, telling our Lord that I was but a humble soldier and to do with me what he willed. "I am here Lord, I come to do your will."

The next several days melded together, half conscious, on the verge of dying, and battling one life-threatening problem after another. The only light at the end of the tunnel came in the form of a rehab center in Colorado called Craig Hospital. I wasn't even sure what would happen there, but I knew it would be a chance to get stronger and a chance to grow into the soldier that our Lord was calling me to be.

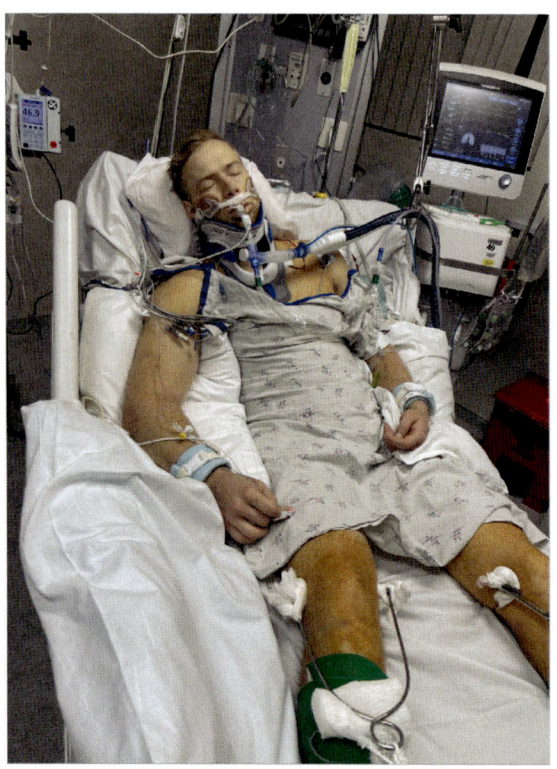

My Mom took this photo to show my father how I looked at the ICU. Notice that my legs were being pulled by brackets screwed into my bones. My wrists were in restraints so I could not pull out my tracheotomy.

Pushing Through the Pain

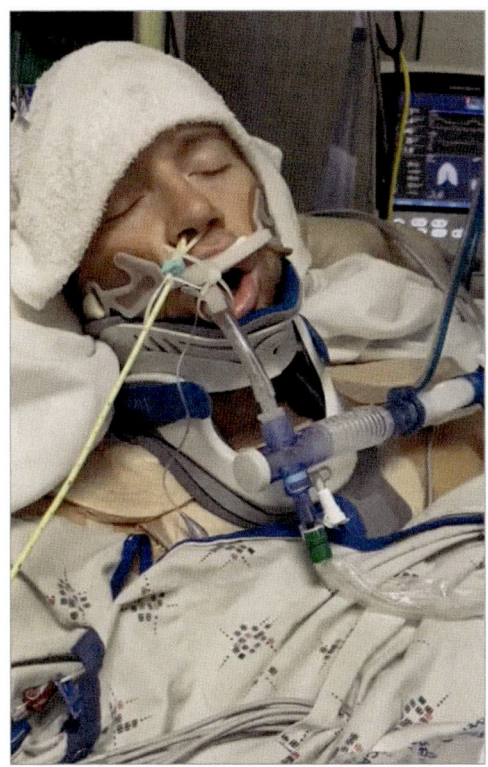

I was on a breathing tube and heavily drugged so I would not bite down on the tube. I suffered immediately from fever and infection.

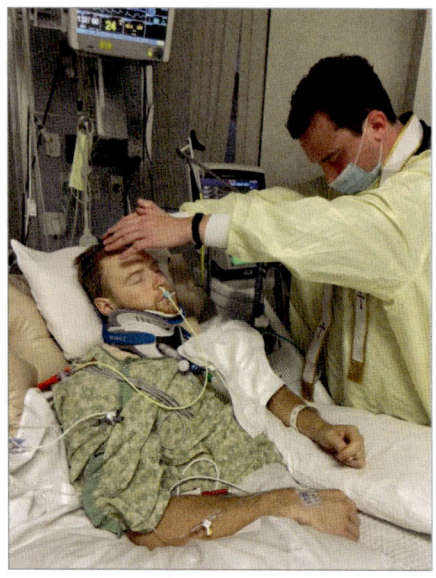

A very good priest came to bring me a blessing and the sacraments.

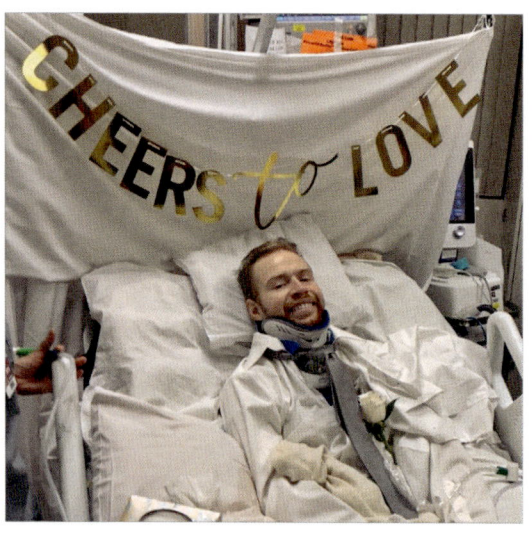

The nurses set me up with a banner, a tie, and a dress shirt for my brother's wedding.

CHAPTER 5

CRAIG HOSPITAL

After forty days and forty nights, they got the go-ahead to transfer me to Craig Hospital in Colorado. In order to transfer, I needed to take a plane. I was taken off my current ventilator and placed on a portable one. Once I switched over onto a portable ventilator, suddenly everything changed. The timing and durations of my breaths were completely scattered, or at least they felt like it. My mind went into sheer panic, and had no idea what was going on, but I felt like I was suffocating, and there was nothing I could do about it. I couldn't speak, I could only struggle as they told me that my numbers looked good, and that I should be fine.

Imagine someone putting their hand over your mouth and plugging your nose. Next, imagine that they get to choose when you get to breathe and for how long. You try to gasp for air, only for it to be too late, the hand is back over your mouth. Imagine the terror of waiting for the next moment that oxygen will come into your lungs, waiting, hoping, praying that it comes before you pass out. That was only the beginning of what it felt like to be on a ventilator.

Then, of course, it felt like a different quality of air being pumped into my lungs, making it hard to feel like I was getting enough air. I'm sure that the actual quality and quantity were carefully measured and were not altered, but I couldn't help but feel like they were different. Both the quantity and quality seemingly changing so rapidly almost sent me into a panic attack. Not only did I feel like I was suffocating, but no one understood and kept just telling me that my numbers looked good, so I shouldn't worry. That was one of the most terrifying experiences I could imagine. I felt like I was dying and everyone just tried to reassure me that I was fine. Although deep down I know they did everything they could for me, it didn't help me deal with the anxiety and worry over the situation

Oftentimes we brush off other people's problems because we assume what it would be like to be in that situation, when the reality is much different. There is so little that we know of what's going on in someone else's life, and the type of suffering that they are enduring. Always be patient and go out of your way to take care of people the way they need to be taken care of, and not just the way that we assume that they should be.

When I finally made it to Craig Hospital, I was in shock. There were so many new faces, so many new surroundings. Once again trach was attached to a new ventilator with new air, it was almost too much and I nearly passed out from anxiety. I waited for my father, knowing how much it would help to have a familiar face but also knowing he would watch over me, speak for me, and advocate for me. Because of Covid restrictions, I had not seen my father since before the accident. I missed him and looked forward to his strength and humor. He was not there on my first day and I could not understand what had happened. I had no way of knowing he had gotten ill while traveling to Colorado and was isolated and suffering alone in a hotel room nearby. Neither of us knew that his texts had never arrived due to cellphone glitches. I was overwhelmed with isolation and feeling lost. I lay in bed, waiting for my father, who was not to come.

The first thing that the doctors did while I was there was run tests and take a couple of x-rays. Included with these x-rays was one of my chest and lungs. For whatever reason, and God knows, one that I will never understand, a black spot appeared on my lung x-ray. This sent the team into overdrive as they were worried that I had contracted tuberculosis. I was immediately packed up and sent into an isolation chamber. A room with no view of the outside world or contact with my parents or anyone I loved. When the nurses or doctors came in to visit me, they were suited up like astronauts or a hazard team. They tried to make me feel comfortable while making me lonelier than I'd ever been. I have never felt so isolated or cut off from humanity. My poor parents, who had only left my side for a couple of hours, came back to find me in total isolation, and all visiting privileges revoked. They were no longer allowed to see me, and they had no idea how long it would last. I waited patiently in the dungeon, still trying to get my bearings and figure out what was going on. It was hard interacting with the nurses when they came in because their faces were disfigured by their suits, and it made them lose all human connection. They truly felt like aliens. They took a follow-up x-ray three days later and noticed that the spot was still there. The medical team identified that there were additional possible reasons why that spot could have appeared and just started to test for tuberculosis directly. The test lasted about a week, and thankfully it came back negative. I did not have tuberculosis. It turns out the spot on my x-ray was from an extremely bad pneumonia infection that I had had earlier.

Finally, I was allowed to move into my own room. They explained that both my parents could visit, though only one at a time because of Covid, I was excited to see my father, whom I had not seen since before my accident. As they brought me in, I was overjoyed to see his tall figure standing in the room waiting for me. It had been so long since I had seen him, and I knew his strength would help me with all that I must do to get strong. However, as soon as he turned to greet me, I saw his face. His face was carved with sorrow and heartbreak. His eyes were worn with worry and grief. His shoulders sagged with the burden of wanting to help and not knowing how. I was overwhelmed and in that moment realized how bad my accident really was. His face was the mirror of truth I had not yet seen. We both paused for a moment, not knowing what to say. And then he rushed to me and hugged me with a mighty grasp that nearly knocked my chair over. Then he stood up straight and said, "Let's get your room set up." I nodded and the practical work of unpacking helped us both snap out of our sorrow. As he unpacked my things, we discussed where to put them. I was allowed pictures on the walls, and other personal items. It was far more than a hospital room. It felt like an apartment. As we worked to make the room feel comfortable, I began to relax. It was a beautiful room, with wide open windows. I could see the sky and the city below me. My father and I were side by side, looking out the far expanse, him standing and I sitting, and we both took a deep breath. We would be ok. We would do this together and I would be ok.

THERE WERE A LOT of young people at Craig Hospital. It seemed like its focus was very much on helping those with otherwise strong bodies to either overcome their injuries or to be able to work with them. There was a big focus on both occupational therapy (how to relearn doing daily tasks with the patient's new limits) and physical therapy (determining what capabilities were possible and making those stronger). I met some amazing young men at this time, and we continue to be friends to this day, encouraging each other and laughing over life's bizarre complications.

But along with my independence from the ICU, came the harsh awareness of my medical situation. I became terribly aware of my feeding tube. This was a tube that ran straight into my stomach. Three times a day a liquid substance was poured down the tube into my stomach. I never felt like I had eaten anything, never felt like I had drunk anything and my mind perceived that I was constantly starving. I lost forty pounds while I was on the feeding tube and felt constantly weak. When it was my mom's turn to visit, she was horrified. She took a picture of me and showed me. I was shocked. My skin color was blue, and I looked terribly emaciated. My mom asked them to give me more food, but they could not because the stomach could not take any more. I felt physically sick, and my stomach was distended, but never full. It was the worst kind of torture. I could not get off the feeding tube until I got off the ventilator, that much I understood. But I had no idea that in the meantime, my body had forgotten how to eat and swallow. I had no idea of the hell that lay before me.

While I could take this time to continue the story of my experience, my suffering, and my life, I feel that it is important to take a step back, to appreciate some of the lessons learned up to this point and highlight what I was able to understand. One of the most important aspects of my journey was learning how to deal with not being in control. We naturally fight to be in complete control of our lives every day, and falsely begin to believe that we in fact have that control. I myself have fallen victim to this mindset and continue to struggle with this notion. While not evil in itself, it becomes a problem when we feel owed a specific outcome from our efforts. Frankly put, we are owed nothing. Even our very existence is not our own. While it is good to strive for the best from this life, we must realize, like Job[1], that everything we have belongs to God. We must let this frame our mindset as we move forward in our lives. Instead of viewing every negative experience and unfortunate circumstance as undeserved and unfair, we ought to view it as carefully crafted by God to help us reflect back on him. Creator over all of the cosmos, he knit us in our mother's womb. He knew that coffee would spill on our shirt before an important interview, that a broken arm would prevent us from playing college football, and that a loved one would die early. These painful life experiences have been woven into a grand tapestry of life before time began. Carefully crafted so that we could live our lives to our fullest potential, bringing sinners to heaven, and glorifying God. Talk

---

1. Job 1:21 "He said, "Naked I came from my mother's womb, and naked shall I return there; the LORD gave, and the LORD has taken away; blessed be the name of the LORD."

about mind blowing. We cannot imagine, or even begin to fathom, the intricacies of our daily lives, and yet, we can know with faith that God has put everything into our lives as it should be.

While it is natural to feel upset or disheartened when our hard work goes unnoticed or doesn't turn out in our favor, it is supernatural faith that guides us into knowing that it is part of God's plan for us and turns us into the perfect creations that we were always meant to be. We have the role of accepting God's grace, and choosing to accept his will for us. That is our sole purpose in this world, this is the only thing that we are called to do every day. That is what will bring us eternal happiness in heaven. This concept is almost impossible for us to understand naturally, but God's grace can give us the strength to endure. His grace will allow us to join with the saints in saying, "If God is with me, who can be against me, for with God all things are possible."

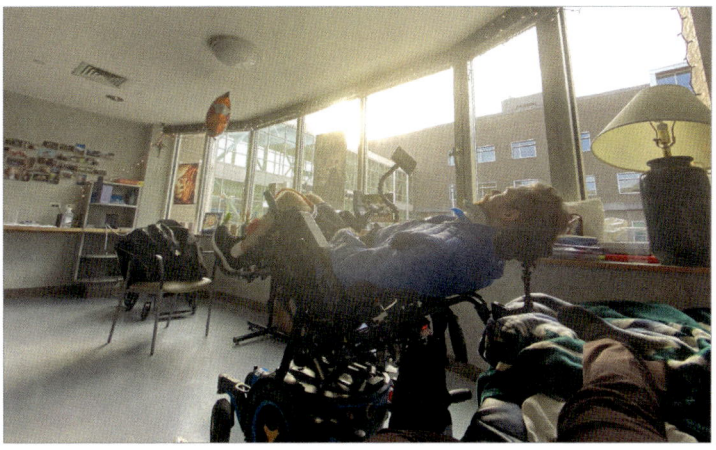

Laying back in the winter sun in my room at Craig Hospital.

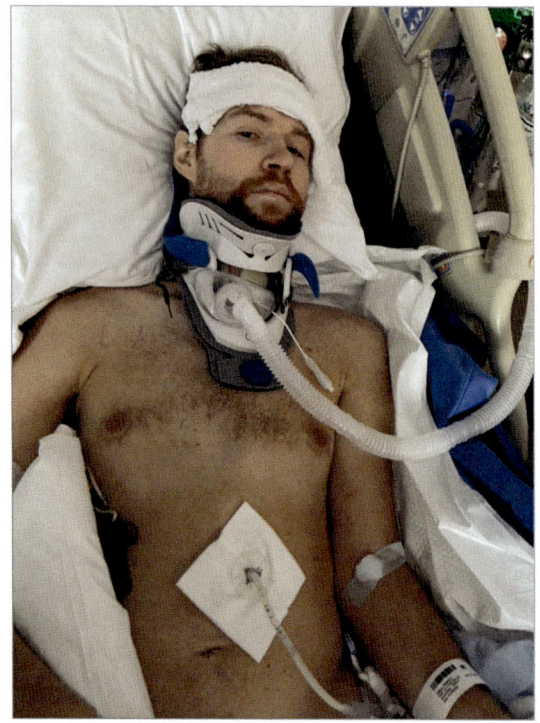

*My mom took this picture because she was so horrified at how much weight I had lost and how depressed I looked.
I was very angry at this picture but she smiled and told me it was a "before photo" so I could see how much I had improved in the "after photo".*

CHAPTER 6

LEARNING TO BREATHE

Recovering from my original trauma of Craig Hospital, I was pounded with a plethora of testing. I had ultrasounds and MRIs, ASIA tests, chest x-rays, and breathing tests. The first week was extremely busy and overwhelming, but somehow, I managed to make it through in good spirits. With all the initial tests completed, I met with the team, and we went over the general goals and schedule of my rehabilitation. One of the first things on my list was learning how to breathe again, a terrifying task that was even harder than I thought, and yet one that seemed so simple.

Let me just tell you, going back to breathing is not like riding a bike. I mentioned before what it was like to be taken off the breathing tube for a short period of time. It's like being underwater, trying to hold your breath, and when you need to breathe you can't take in any air. Your body doesn't physically pass out, but your mind feels like it should. Caught in this loop of torture and never-ending suffocation. You start off with five minutes, five minutes of not breathing air. Just barely kept alive, struggling desperately to tell your body that it should be able to do this on its own. You want to scream and wake your body up; a task that you never had thought about before is a task that you can no longer do and have no control over. You desperately try to remember what it feels like, anything that can help you ignite those muscles so that you can breathe again. And yet, still nothing, you can't control it like you do an arm or leg, your body just breathes; and so it seems impossible to help your body succeed. How the heck am I supposed to do this, I wonder. Five minutes have gone by, and I tap out, my anxiety through the roof, and I feel like my airways have been shut the whole time with just a little bit of air sneaking in and out. I can't imagine that I will ever be able to do this again, let alone for the rest of my life. I despair a little but decide to let that be tomorrow's problem and not let it consume me today.

Tomorrow comes. I double down on my efforts, convincing myself that I can do better. I ask the respiratory therapist for help, using only a few words with the breaths that I have available. He tells me that the most important key to unlocking the ability to breathe is consistency. He explains that the breathing muscles, namely the diaphragm, is so thin that it loses capability within twenty-four hours if not continually utilized. But by the same token, it builds up again, just as fast, and as long as you don't let it forget its previous progress, you'll notice a great increase in your capabilities. He tells me this might feel impossible, but if every time I focus on breathing as long as I can, take no more than a quick break and do it over again, that before I know it, I'll be breathing normally again. His words sound crazy, as none of this is registering in my brain other than as a hopeful fantasy. However, deep down, my background in medicine is telling me that what he is saying makes sense, and that it's worth giving it a shot. I prepare for the worst and let go of the ventilator as I spin off into the darkness, fighting to breathe.

Time ticks slowly by, one minute after another, as I still cannot overcome the feeling that I am slowly suffocating. I keep pushing forward, constantly looking back at the clock, painfully aware of the slow progress. I make it fifteen minutes this time, once again on the verge of giving up for the day. I feel like all of my fighting investments are pointless. Once again, the respiratory therapist doubles down, telling me to take a quick break, and then try again. I am exhausted, anxious, and feel it is impossible for me to do better, let alone try again. Deep down within me, I promise myself that if I try two more times, I can call it for the day. I set my jaw once again and give the signal to stop the ventilator. I fight with every ounce of my being to do better than my previous record. I somehow manage to make it to thirty minutes before tapping out again. I am impressed. But I feel the strain of the extra work, and I'm not convinced that it was any easier. I break for ten minutes and go again, this time only making it to twenty minutes. Somehow, this still doesn't seem like it's working for me. I collapse, exhausted and tired. I can't do it anymore. The respiratory therapist says that I did a good job, and he'll come back and check on me toward the end of the day.

There's a knock on the door. I come to my senses, not sure how long it's been, not sure if I've been sleeping or just zoned out. I look at the clock, it's been several hours, I must've passed out after the hard work this morning. The respiratory therapist steps into the room, comes over to me, and says, "Are you ready to start again?" Dumbfounded, I stare back at him with a look clearly saying,

"No effing way. You've got to be kidding me. Can't you see how exhausted I am?"

There was no way I felt up to doing it again. He just looked at me and assured me that the work I did that morning would make a difference if I continued, but if I rested any longer, all of those muscles that I gained would disappear. It made no sense; how could the small effort I put in this morning actually make a difference in my muscles? How could I lose it in just another eight hours? My head was still spinning, and I braced myself as I knew what I must do, what I had to do. I gave him a nod, and again he took me off the ventilator.

I bared my teeth, convinced that this was going to suck so much more. I was convinced that I would only make it ten minutes before tapping out. But as I closed my eyes and clenched my teeth, time started to pass. I kept waiting for that moment of exhaustion, but my body started to find its stride; the effort of breathing didn't seem to hit me the same way. Unbelievably, I cracked my eyes open to look at the clock, convinced that, somehow, no time had passed. But the clock confirmed what my body was saying: it had already been half an hour, and I felt like I had just started. I kept going. How could it be this easy? Was it a miracle? Is that really how science works? I didn't question it anymore; I simply continued to breathe. Before long, an hour had passed, and the respiratory therapist was telling me that I had to go back to the ventilator. What? I couldn't believe it. I didn't even have to tap out. I was told to take a break. I agreed, still somewhat shocked about what had just happened. He once again told me that the diaphragm muscles grow and disappear in such a short time that if you put in the work, you can see so much change in less than a day.

Suddenly, it started to click; in the past, I had just given up and come back to it the next day. But by then, the muscle had disappeared, and I was back to square one all over again. An hour passed, and the respiratory therapist asked if I wanted to go again. I was excited. I agreed, curious to see if this theory held up, and if I would be able to last even longer than before. Sure enough, my muscles kicked back into gear and my diaphragm started working. This time I made it two hours before he told me I needed to go back to the ventilator. Except this time, I didn't want to go back. My body realized what it was supposed to be doing and now felt trapped going back to the ventilator. It was like being told when you can breathe and when you can't. The ventilator, which had given me life just moments before, now felt like a torture device. I asked if I could just keep going using my diaphragm. He said I had to go back to the ventilator to make sure I didn't over exhaust my muscles. I hesitantly agreed, trusting again in the wisdom of the therapist. I was so excited that my muscles were doing what they were supposed to and I couldn't wait to be independent from the ventilator.

However, after a couple of hours on the ventilator, I started to get massive anxiety. I asked to go back to normal breathing. The pattern of the ventilator no longer made sense. I was fully aware of the need to control my own breathing. They allowed me to go off the ventilator, and this time I lasted four hours before they wanted me to go back on it again. I expressed my concern and asked if there was any other way. They told me that I was already jumping through hoops and skipping steps. Typically, they were a lot more strict, and the time frames were a lot more narrow for when people are allowed to go without the ventilator.

Begrudgingly, I eventually conceded, while at the same time discussing with the doctor how many more shifts of the ventilator I would have to do before I could cut it off completely. After a little more back and forth, we came up with a plan, and the timeline was set, and I would be completely off the ventilator in a little over a week. It was amazing how something could change so fast and go from a life-giving stream to an absolute nightmare. The hours that I had to spend on the ventilator were excruciating. My anxiety was through the roof as they plugged me into the machine when my body knew that it could breathe on its own. The time that I needed on the ventilator gradually changed and lessened and eventually faded away. The freedom of breathing on my own was intoxicating, and it felt like the first real step in my recovery. Being able to talk, communicate, and breathe all of my own volition brought me so much hope, and strength to persevere and push on. Strength that I would greatly need moving forward, for I did not know all of the battles that lay before me.

Although I had been weaned off the ventilator, they needed to keep my trach in for another two weeks because my diaphragm was not strong enough to cough up all of the mucus that my body produced. The trach was a hole in my throat that went straight to my lungs, previously allowing the ventilator to provide my lungs with oxygen. Now that I was off the ventilator, they would plug the trach to allow my lungs to function on their own. However when my lungs became overwhelmed with mucus and prevented me from breathing, they needed to stick a vacuum down my trach and suction it out. This transition, while being forward progress and something I was very proud of, brought with it a whole slew of complications. It also showed me that the road to recovery was going to be long, and there were no easy or quick fixes to getting better. I knew that my patience would be tested. So much suffering and difficulty lay in store for me, some that I knew about and much that I would only find out later. There was nowhere to go but forward, so I gritted my teeth, steadied my emotions, and pushed forward into the dark, not knowing what lay in store but responding to our Lord's call: "Take up your cross and follow me."

Patience comes in two forms, either waiting for something when we know it will be given to us or having hope for something we cannot see or may not receive. For so much of my life, most of my experience with patience had to do with knowing what would happen but just having to wait for it, like a kid excited for presents on Christmas, or looking forward to summer break. Most of my recovery had been the other sort: being forced to persevere and endure without knowing what the future held in store. I was forced to take each hurdle and trial as it came. I had to trust that God knew what I could bear and would always provide me with enough grace to see it through. I took great consolation by meditating on examples in the Bible. The first being Jesus himself, knowing what must happen while still maintaining the course and patiently waiting for it to come about. The second being the example of Job, who had to wait without knowing why or when his suffering would end.

From that time on, Jesus began to show his disciples that he must go to Jerusalem and undergo great suffering at the hands of the elders and chief priests and scribes, and be killed, and on the third day be raised. And Peter took him aside and began to rebuke him, saying, "God forbid it, Lord! This must never happen to you." But he turned and said to Peter, "Get behind me, Satan! You are a stumbling block to me; for you are setting your mind not on divine things but on human things" (Matthew 16:21–23).

Jesus understood the need for his sacrifice and refused to entertain the idea of not going through with it. He patiently waited for God's perfect timing to bring about his crucifixion and death.

Meanwhile, Job had no idea what was in store for him but knew that he must persevere and trust that God was in control:

> God gives me up to the ungodly,
> and casts me into the hands of the wicked.
> I was at ease, and he broke me in two;
> he seized me by the neck and dashed me to pieces;
> he set me up as his target;
> His archers surround me.
> He slashes open my kidneys, and shows no mercy;
> he pours out my gall on the ground.
> He bursts upon me again and again;
> he rushes at me like a warrior.
> I have sewed sackcloth upon my skin,
> and have laid my strength in the dust.
> My face is red with weeping,
> and deep darkness is on my eyelids,
> though there is no violence in my hands,
> and my prayer is pure. (Job 16:11–17)

This is Job's cry to our Lord in the midst of his suffering, not understanding why it is brought about, yet despite all the suffering he endures he never curses the Lord. In the New Testament, James commends Job, praising him for enduring all the suffering that God has allowed upon him: "Indeed, we call blessed those who showed endurance. You have heard of the endurance of Job, and you have seen the purpose of the Lord, how the Lord is compassionate and merciful" (James 5:11).

Throughout our lives, we will experience a call for patience. Whether or not we're put into the situation of Job or our Lord, we must respond with our Lord: "Not my will, but your will be done."

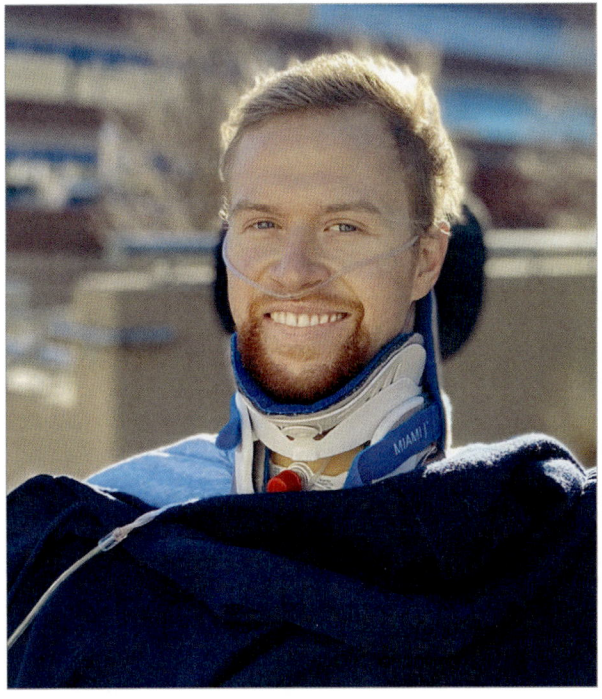

I was so happy to be free from the ventilator and go outside.

CHAPTER 7

DAILY LIFE PARALYZED

As I got more comfortable breathing on my own, the doctor told me that I would be participating more actively in PT (physical therapy) and OT (occupational therapy). I didn't know what this meant until I was woken up early in the morning and told to meet at the gym in an hour. Oh, the gym. Just the word brings back so many memories of myself before the accident. So much time, so much work, so many strong emotions. I loved working out, feeling the stretch of my muscles, feeling the sweat gather and fall down my face. Pushing myself to the point of exertion and then just a little bit further. The satisfaction of seeing my hard work pay off. The many friendships that I made along the way formed by a common goal. Would the gym ever be the same? Would I ever have those feelings again?

I pondered all of these thoughts in the back of my head as I began the hourlong routine of getting ready in the morning. The entire process began with stretching. Because my body does not move during the night, when I wake up, all of my muscles are stiff. In order to make sure that I got proper blood flow, fought off spasms, and stayed flexible, I needed to stretch. Typically, this was around fifteen to twenty minutes and generally involved manipulating my legs to help free the tendons and loosen up the muscles. The next step was a bed bath to make sure I had no lingering bacteria on my body that could cause any kind of infection or problem throughout the day. While I was getting a bed bath, the nurses made sure to check for any pressure wounds or skin irritations to help prevent a breakdown of my skin or any kind of internal bruising. I already had a pressure wound on my tailbone that they were watching. It was a small reminder of the time in the ICU, lying on my back for so long. Even though the nurses had worked so hard to turn me and relieve that pressure, a small wound began. They put healing salves on it and carefully bandaged it to help protect it. It was interesting to me that they used silver-infused bandages which help fight bacteria. At home my mom had used a silver spray to help with the healing of animals. And though the animals all healed from various mishaps, some more serious than others, we never knew if the practice was just a placebo or if it really worked. It was great to see that the most advanced hospitals in America were also using silver to fight bacteria and help with the healing.

The final step was to attach a leg bag so that urine could drain into it throughout the day. Since I could not urinate normally, I had a catheter placed through my abdomen directly into my bladder, which ran down my leg and then connected to the leg bag. Finally, I was ready to get dressed. This meant a lot of rolling side to side as the nurse wrestled different articles of clothing up my legs and into the proper positions. After underwear, pants, socks, and shoes, I was finally ready for the last step—the binder. I wore an abdominal binder that helped regulate my blood pressure because I did not have any core strength. It helped keep the blood from just sitting in my gut and causing my blood pressure to dip and me to pass out. This binder also helped keep my stomach and intestines compressed so that blood could flow more easily to my extremities. Now that the binder was on, I was ready to be transferred with a sling into my chair.

The sling is an interesting contraption. It is basically a flat piece of strong material with loops or handles on each corner. They turned me on my side, and tucked the long cloth under my body, then rolled my body back over the cloth. Then they hooked the loops onto a hoist and slowly raised the arm of the hoist. This had the effect of folding the cloth and my body into a seated position. This way they could lift me from the bed into my wheelchair. My family came to enjoy using one of these like a game, as they would have one slinging me and my siblings around the room. But at the time, it felt utterly humiliating, like I was a piece of meat at a butcher store.

Once I was in my chair, the nurses helped me with a shirt and helped adjust me in the chair so that my posture was good. All of the turning from getting dressed had loosened up mucus from my lungs. So before I headed out, the nurses suctioned out my lungs and cleared any mucus clots, so I didn't accidentally choke and pass out. I still could not eat or drink, so this was the extent of my routine in the morning. The whole process took over forty minutes, and I was already exhausted, just in time to go to the gym. I rolled my eyes internally; the irony hurt just a little bit more than I cared to admit. I then finally headed to my appointment in the gym.

I didn't know what to expect. I had always loved going to the gym and working out with fellow gym members, encouraging each other, and enjoying the feeling of getting stronger. As we rolled in, I saw a bunch of empty wheelchairs on the side and rows of elevated mats with men and women struggling, each in their own way. I tried to ignore the empty eyes and bodies falling over. I tried to ignore the tortured look of parents and loved ones along the wall, watching with forced smiles and hollow encouraging words. I focused on the fact that I was here to get strong and, like any other challenge I had faced, I would do my best to succeed.

I wondered what the plan would be. I was excited to get to work as I'd been lying in bed for so long, and a part of me felt good to finally start doing something. I tapered my expectations, knowing that I was extremely limited in what I was able to do and would be easily frustrated at just how limited my capabilities were. I did my best to push all of my emotions aside and focus on simply exceeding the expectations placed on me by my therapists.

The first thing we did was make introductions and get a general tour of the gym to orient me. I asked my physical therapist what the plan was for the day, and she informed me that we would try to do some work on the mat but assured me that we would take it slow. I nodded in agreement, still not knowing what that entailed. After a couple of minutes of setup, I got the go-ahead signal and headed over. A giant sling was ready to pick me up and help transfer me onto the mat. The sling was designed in such a way as to go under each leg and behind the back and then lift up. Unfortunately, as the sling lifted me up, there was no longer tension on my butt and combined with the stress of a new situation, I immediately crapped my pants. I couldn't feel anything, so I wasn't sure, but the smell made it pretty easy to put two and two together. I'd never been so embarrassed and humiliated in my entire life. Not only did I crap my pants but now I needed to ask my physical therapist to check and see if I did. She didn't hesitate to jump right in and help me out, trying to make the awkward situation feel as normal as possible, but I was still mortified. She got a glove, did a quick check and let me know that I had in fact crapped myself. Distraught, I hung my head low as she explained that I would be taken back to my bed to get everything squared away. I was at a loss for words; I didn't even have the opportunity to be alone to express it. I buried it deep inside, removed myself from reality, and waited for it to be over. My mind didn't even let me think about it, because I knew I would come up with nothing.

I was angry at God. I could think of no good reason that I should have to crap my pants in addition to dealing with everything else going on. It felt like a sick joke and cruel humor. I tried to think of our Lord, and his humility. I was trying desperately to find some parallel between our situations. All of my examples seemed to come up empty, I had never read in the Bible about Jesus crapping his pants. What was I supposed to turn to for consolation? In the back of my head, this question kept turning, trying to make sense of something that seemed so ridiculous. Jesus was the king of humility, why couldn't I find a similarity? I prayed more deeply and reflected further on the humility of Jesus, and the Holy Spirit guided me and helped put me in my place.

Jesus, who is God, became man. What simple words that we repeat in the Creed so often as Catholics and yet think about so little. God, who is infinitely greater than us in every way, was willing to limit himself by such a profound margin by taking on a human body. He took on the confines and natural laws that constrict a human body. We enter the world as humans and live our lives bound by the body. We do not perceive eliminating waste as a humiliating and degrading thing. But God took on that humility, knowing what it was like not to be bound by the body and its functions. God becoming man is infinitely more humiliating to him, than it is for us to be reduced to a pile of crap. How dare I look at my own situation in life, and think that I held a candle to Jesus's humility? What a realization. It helped put my mind at ease and refocus on my priorities. It gave me strength to keep pushing forward, regardless of how many times I crapped my pants. Although I knew I would never be able to understand the depths of our Lord's humility, I could at least take solace in knowing that my own struggles were nothing compared to his, and that by uniting my humility to our Lord's, I would be able to grow closer to him.

The day ended with my ego feeling pretty beaten, and I thought to myself that things couldn't get worse, so it was all up from here. I closed my eyes and tried to visualize the next day and the progress that would surely come from it.

The next few days were a blur—a tiring, exhausting, and humiliating blur. But each day I felt like I was making progress. Coughing up a little more phlegm, getting stronger, working out and stretching. But as the days passed, I waited anxiously to learn how to eat. I fantasized about food and remembered the days of eating a hamburger with tears in my eyes. It had been over fifty days since I had eaten any food. Or drank water for that matter. I dreamed of water and rain, longing for that feeling of coolness on my parched throat.

Before I was allowed to eat, they had to take the trach out of my throat, and in order to do that, they had to stop suctioning my lungs to clear mucus buildup. They explained to me that this was all a normal part of the healing process, and my lungs and muscles just needed to get stronger so that I could have the endurance and strength to cough up the mucus myself. I acknowledged their wisdom, as I knew they had probably seen this time and time again. I remained patient and continued pushing myself and working hard.

After many more days in the gym, and unfortunately several more accidents, they told me that I could take the next step in rehab, which was to cap off my trach for three days and see if my body could fight off mucus buildup on its own. My trach was given a red cap. This was an incredible moment. I was not only fully separated from the breathing machine, but that red cap was a sign to all the world that I could breathe on my own. If I made it three days without needing any help, then I could get the tube pulled out permanently and work toward eating.

At first, I was riddled with anxiety, this was a big step, and I wasn't sure if my body was ready for it. To aid with the transition I always had someone around me so that if I needed to clear mucus from my throat, they could just give me the Heimlich maneuver to help me cough it out. This was an intermediary step, so that I was not completely on my own, but all of the help was purely external. My mom and I had taken lifeguard classes together, along with most of my siblings, so she had a rough (and I do mean rough) idea of the Heimlich method. I was able to show her how to use both hands, flat out, to push against the lower part of my lungs to push out mucus. She got pretty good at it, and one time while at the gym, I nodded to her and she pushed heavily, practically popping the mucus out of my mouth. The nurses were at first worried and then impressed that she not only didn't hurt me, but that we had gotten the mucus out so effectively.

I quickly learned that I could just double over when I really needed to get a strong compression to hack up the mucus in my lungs. The time that it was the most difficult was during the night when gravity was against me, and I couldn't move. I lay in my bed trying to hack up mucus for half an hour before finally calling the nurses for help so that they could help compress my lungs and get the mucus out. This woke me up every hour or two, causing me severe lack of sleep and lots of mental anguish. Fears about whether this would always be my life crept in and haunted me.

Even though I still needed assistance, the three required days finally passed, and as promised, they scheduled an appointment to get the tube taken out of my throat. What had so long been a source of irritation and a reminder of all the trauma I had been through was finally getting purged from my body. Although I had functionally been living without it, the idea of it being completely removed felt momentous, marking a major milestone in my recovery. However, the removal was not nearly as dramatic as I imagined. With a simple three-two-one, they pulled it out and a bandage was placed over the hole. Amazing how simple and yet life-changing that moment was. The bandage sealed the hole in my throat so that no air could escape. I immediately felt the change, my airway felt so much more open, and it gave me a sense of pride knowing that my body was fighting on its own. My airways were finally clear. I was breathing on my own, and nothing was in the way. This was clearly how our body was meant to be. The air had never felt so fresh. I was told that the healing would take a little over a week, and then I could start working on eating and drinking again. I was happy and proud of my achievements and excited to start the next stage of recovery. However, though

I had won the battle of breathing on my own, I had no idea that the war was far from over.

As I waited for the hole in my throat to close, I spent more time in therapy working on functional skills and strength. It felt good to feel my body strengthening the muscles that I had for so long ignored; however, it was equally as difficult to realize that there were some muscles I would never get back, no matter how hard I tried. My abs, which had once been a symbol of my hours committed to the gym, and my athletic strength, were now reduced to a pouch of internal organs splayed out from my abdomen, vulnerable and exposed. Those muscles, which no longer had life, were a constant cross and reminder of everything that had happened and the fragility of our bodies. My vanity was shattered, knowing that even the most intense dedication would not cover such an obvious flaw. These thoughts entered my brain, but I pushed them back, realizing that beyond mere appearance I had also lost functionality by losing those muscles, something a hundred times more important. This was another wave of sorrow, more intense than the last as I knew that not having these muscles dramatically limited everything I could do. It is so easy to assume that life in a wheelchair simply involves the inability to walk, when in reality that is the least of the problems. Without internal core strength, one cannot sit, one cannot balance, and one cannot circulate blood effectively, just to name a few problems. It is fascinating and depressing to realize how much work the strength of the body's core does to help the body function.

I brushed aside my self-pity, and once again set my jaw and doubled down to strengthen what I did have, not letting my mind go down the rabbit hole of loss and what used to be. Every workout felt different, strange, and surreal, as even the simplest movement became a balancing act as my body couldn't hold itself up to resist the workouts. Every time I did an arm curl, my body wanted to flop down onto the ground. It was a balancing game, without having any of the tools to balance. It was like trying to balance a set of scales except every time I tried to balance them, someone flicked the scales with their finger. This was not at all what working out used to be; irritation and anger boiled inside of me as I realized that this would be the future of working out.

All I could do was push forward and fight like hell. As I worked out, I looked around at the faces of everyone else struggling with the same reality. Never had I seen such emptiness, so many people in shell shock, stunned in disbelief. Each of us fighting our own battles, while trying to hold on to a shred of dignity as we asked for help for every little thing. I wish I had the words to embolden each of them, to give them hope and strength to keep fighting, but words failed me, and my own cloud of darkness prevented me from finding the strength to even speak. The best I could do was to push myself and hope that by my example they would be able to garner some strength to persevere and keep fighting. Any of my attempts to encourage people seemed to be empty and fall on deaf ears, as words could not heal the damage done. Only time, perseverance, and faith could fight the despair so manifest in that hospital. I prayed to God that maybe somehow my example would help others find strength, as I felt that my words could not.

The phrase "actions speak louder than words" is very near and dear to my heart. I have always felt strongly that we must be examples of faith in our lives and not just talk about it. As it says in the Bible, "you will know them by their fruits"

Matt 7, 2. We watch and see what people do, and how they act in order to know if they believe. How easy it is to say one thing and do another. Or to make exceptions for ourselves. We tell ourselves that if we were just in another situation, we would be able to act virtuously. When the reality is, we are always given the grace to choose what's right, regardless of our situation. We must fight for the strength not to give in or give up. We are often quick to judge, but slow to act. That is why actions speak so strongly of someone's character, because while it is easy to say something, it is hard to do it.

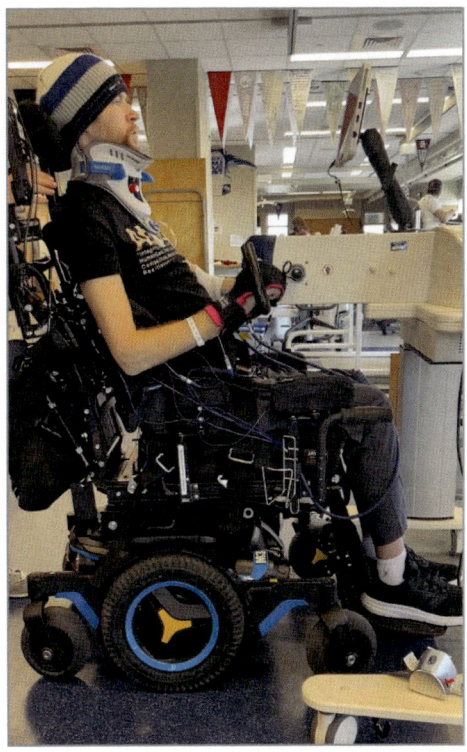

Part of my Physical Therapy was "bicycling" with my arms to not only increase strength but to help with my blood circulation. Notice the loss of muscle in my arms from when I was first in the ICU.

CHAPTER 8

THE PROBLEM OF FOOD

I pushed myself to work out every day, gradually finding ways to make it more independent—just to carve out one small part of my life that I could truly call my own. Working out felt so good, not just for my mind but also for my health, strengthening my lungs and helping pump blood throughout my body. I have no doubt that this made time pass quickly, and before I knew it, another big step in my journey had finished. The hole in my throat had healed and the doctors gave me permission to start learning how to eat and drink again.

How long I had waited for this day. It seemed like it would never come. All day long I lay in the hospital bed back at the ICU and dreamt about food and water. Since the first day of my accident, all of my food had been delivered through a tube into my stomach. I hadn't tasted food or water for over two months. Water, especially, had been sorely missed, especially with the dry climate in Colorado. I dreamt of guzzling gallons of water or eating a cereal bowl of ice cubes and water, only to wake up dismayed that it was just a dream.

Finally, as silly as they were, my dreams were now coming true. I met with the speech therapist and was excited to get started. She sat down, talked with me and helped prepare me for the journey still to come. She informed me that, just like it was a struggle to breathe again, so also the muscles in the throat would take a while to function properly again. There was a serious danger of inhaling food and water, which could cause a bronchial infection, and even death. I didn't really make much of her warning, as eating and drinking were such a mindless task before my accident that it seemed impossible it would be any different now. However, as with breathing, I was quickly brought back to reality. The first sip of water, that longed-for sip of heaven, brought only horror. It was awful. My body didn't know what it was doing, some water was going down my throat and some was going straight into my lungs. My eyes started watering, and I started a weak cough, trying to get out the water that should've gone down my throat.

Once again it was hard for me to accept this new reality, and fight all over again for something that should be so simple. The thing that I craved for so long was causing me so much difficulty and pain. Every time I took a bite, I tried to swallow, but only the muscles in my mouth cooperated, whereas the muscles in my throat were like an elevator that was mistimed, going up and down but never when the passengers were trying to get on or off. This resulted in a jumbled chaos of food being pushed everywhere, back into my mouth, down my throat, or into my lungs. I kept battling, trying to stick to mushy foods that could go down on their own. Swallowing still never felt right, but my therapist kept telling me that the more I practiced the better it would be. I kept trying. The amazing taste of food and water helped me to keep coming back to it. Every two weeks, after practicing, they took me to the radiology department, where they had me swallow things covered in radio-opaque fluids and keep track of anything that went down the wrong pipe, and whether or not my swallowing was improving.

The first time I took this test it was terrifying. We went down a long hallway into a dark corridor and into what seemed like a prison. It was so dark inside there, with only the glow of several x-ray machines to light the way. Although the plan seemed straightforward, the entire process felt straight out of a horror movie. They had me wheel onto a giant X on the floor and lock my wheelchair. Feeling very much like I had a target on my chest, they placed a heavy leaded vest on me. My speech therapist turned away toward the counter and I was half expecting her to come back with a saw threatening to cut off an appendage if I didn't tell her government secrets. Thankfully that was not the case, but nonetheless she turned around with a cup that I could barely see and offered me a spoonful of some amorphous blob that I could swear was almost glowing from radiation. As I ate, the plan was to run an x-ray video of my throat, recording my swallowing process

I felt pressured to eat it quickly so that my body didn't take on too much radiation from the constant x-rays from the machine, but because it was so dark, I couldn't distinguish what I was eating, and that didn't help convince my mind that I should swallow it. My imagination, coupled with the pressure of knowing this test would determine whether the next two weeks would be enjoyable or more struggling, made it near impossible to perform well. Needless to say, I choked, both figuratively and literally. They moved on to several more items including drinking water from a straw, and eating what I assume was graham cracker and yogurt, but everything felt wrong, and I could tell that it wasn't going well. I left feeling defeated and slightly traumatized.

Moments later, I got the official word that I had not passed the test and was not ready to eat on my own. Although the test was not a wholly accurate representation, I knew it was the truth. I knew I wasn't ready. Whenever I ate, it was all I could do to get the food to go down the right pipe. The coordination of my muscles was all over the map and although I'd already been practicing for two weeks, I could not discern any difference or improvement in my swallowing. It was depressing once again feeling like no matter how hard I worked or what I did, my body did not cooperate with me and it seemed like there was nothing I could do to change that.

This brings me to another point that is very important to me—helplessness. More specifically, being helpless even when you know that everything is happening the way it should. I believe this is the helplessness that God asks us to cultivate in our daily lives by leaning on him. We want so badly to be in control, to have our lives figured out, and to know what the future holds. However, as much as we have figured out, we will never be able to plan for everything and life will keep throwing curveballs. We must not get disheartened when things don't go our way, because this is a good thing. It is a reminder that it is okay not to be in control.

Therefore, do not be anxious, saying "What shall we eat?" or "What shall we drink?" or "What shall we wear?" For the Gentiles seek all these things; and your heavenly Father knows that you need them all. But seek first his kingdom and his righteousness, and all these things shall be yours as well. Therefore, do not be anxious about tomorrow, for tomorrow will be anxious for itself. Let the day's own trouble be sufficient for the day (Matthew 6:31–34).

Jesus is clearly telling us that we can trust in him and not worry about being in control of what happens in our lives. Although we must always strive to make the most out of our lives and do what we can with what God has given us, we must always cultivate the opportunities God gives us to be helpless and call our minds back to our trust in him. A saying that I have always loved and has always been in my life and in my heart is this: "Do the best with what you have and leave the rest to God." God wants us to need him. He wants us to realize that without him we have nothing. We are ultimately in control of nothing, except responding to the grace he gives us to live out our lives every day.

I didn't let discouragement get the best of me, and continued to fight, every day, straining my mind and my muscles and praying that they would work together in unison. I could feel improvement, but it wasn't as fast as I was hoping. Practicing consisted of working with my speech therapist to swallow soft food like pudding or Jell-O and then having her give me feedback as she examined how my muscles attempted to swallow the food. She would give me exercises to practice on my own, like swallowing water continuously through a straw without breathing as long as I could. Or different mouth exercises to strengthen different parts of the swallowing muscles. While the exercises felt like they were working, my body still seemed to struggle with the idea of coordinating everything together. My throat and esophagus were so uncoordinated that I felt like a seagull, regurgitating my food with almost every swallow to prevent it from going into my lungs.

Two more weeks passed by, and it was time to retest my swallowing ability. This time I knew the routine, and I knew what to expect. I was nervous again, and, although I felt like I would do better, I knew there was still probably a fifty-fifty chance I would swallow food down the wrong pipe. I went down to the testing area, put on the lead apron, and began to eat and drink what they put in front of me. It was hard for me to concentrate on chewing and swallowing. I was not confident and was doing everything I could to hold off coughing or tearing up. I just focused on making sure everything went down the right pipe. When they finally told me I was done, I was sure I had failed the test again, and I mentally prepared myself for that reality. It was hard not to feel like it was an impossible task, and that I was never going to be able to overcome it. Once again, I went back to my room and waited for the official decision.

It was at least several hours before I heard anything, which was already a bad sign. Both my speech therapist and my doctor came into the room, looking very somber. When I saw the doctor, I began to get even more nervous, because he only talked to me when there was something serious. They looked at me solemnly and before the doctor began, the nurse rushed in before him and said, "You failed the test. I'm sorry." I lay in my bed, discouraged to the core of my heart. I wanted so badly to eat and drink. I wanted so badly to succeed. However, I felt their presence and looked up. They were not done. What more could possibly be said?

And then the doctor spoke. And in that moment I realized the news of failing the test was not the bad news. The bad news was still coming. The room began to spin with dread as the doctor spoke. "We found a hole in the back of your throat. The metal brace put in your spine after your accident is piercing through into your esophagus. Food is getting caught there and if it enters your spine could cause an infection…." I listened in horror as he continued.

"The situation is serious, and without emergency surgery, you could go septic and be dead within several days."

Their words fell on deaf ears, as I could barely process what they were saying. I nodded to show recognition while slowly retreating into myself. They kept talking, telling me that it was a miracle nothing had gotten stuck in there already and caused an infection. They then explained that surgery would be the best option to repair the hole and briefly went over the details of what had to happen next. I'm sure they could see my disengagement, and so they made it brief and told me they would schedule the surgery within a few days.

As miraculous as it was that they found it, the news was devastating. Not only was I not going to be able to eat on my own, but I wasn't going to be able to eat or drink anything for at least a month. I was expressionless. I was completely dumbstruck. I was crushed and didn't know who to blame. I prayed quietly to our Lord, asking him why he had put me through this after everything I had already been through. Had I not already suffered enough? This just felt cruel. However, I offered it up once again saying, "I am your servant, Lord, if this is your will, then I will do it even if I take no enjoyment in it." Just as a soldier marches into battle, knowing the profound suffering, pain, and even death that he might face, so I also continued to hold fast trusting that our Lord knew what he was doing.

What lay before me felt insurmountable. In preparation for the surgery, what little food and water I was allowed to consume would be taken away from me, what little progress I had made would disappear. I had been working so hard to get stronger in the gym, and now I would be bedridden for a month recovering from surgery, and I knew that all of my muscles would atrophy all over again and going back would feel the same as the first day. The reality of my situation felt surreal, straight out of a nightmare where I had to relive one of the worst months of my life. I cannot even describe how devastating a blow it was. My mind went numb with disbelief. There was nothing I could do to avoid it. I couldn't run and disappear. There was nothing that could distract me from the enormous suffering that lay before me. Once again, I turned to God, accepting the suffering, albeit begrudgingly, and just left everything else up to him. One of the hardest things was giving up the ability to drink water. It was something that I had cherished so much since I had been deprived of it for so long. The cold, arid climate of the high deserts in Colorado made my mouth immediately dry up and kept me awake at night for lack of moisture. The only thing that they allowed me to do was to dampen my mouth with a sponge, which felt as pointless as watering the desert with a watering can. I couldn't help thinking of our Lord on the cross calling out to the soldiers saying, "I thirst," and then being given a sponge soaked with wine. "At once one of them ran and got a sponge, filled it with sour wine, put it on a stick, and gave it to him to drink" (Matthew 27:48).

The day of surgery finally arrived, and the reality of what was going to transpire was sinking in. I was suddenly terrified they would put me on a ventilator, and I would be stuck with it, once again, trapped and unable to breathe. I reached out to the doctor and begged him not to leave me on it. He stopped and looked at me, his matter-of-fact eyes suddenly filled with compassion. He shook his head and said, "No ventilator. You will wake up breathing on your own." This gave me some consolation.

The plan was to cut open my throat so they could patch

a hole in my esophagus and then sew it back together. There was a chance it could compromise my ability to swallow permanently. I said a prayer, and once again offered my life to our Lord, knowing that everything was in his hands, and all of this was according to his plan. I was wheeled into the hospital room, the gas mask put on, and within just a few moments, my eyes shut, and my mind turned off.

I woke up over thirteen hours later after an intense surgery. I was in a foreign room, unable to speak and in pain. I was terrified. With Covid still in full force, visitations were limited, if not completely impossible. I closed my eyes, and tried to pretend that it was all over, and that I no longer had to endure the suffering. Yet try as I might, I was still very present and aware of my intense pain. I held fast with stubborn determination, continually saying to myself that I would make it through this and offering it up to our Lord. Yet even as I prayed, the words sounded so repetitive and hollow it was hard to feel that they meant anything. And yet, I knew that simply earnestly saying the words was enough, even if I felt no consolation from them.

The next three weeks were awful, each day slower than the next, with nothing to do except lie in bed and dream about food and water. They wouldn't let me eat or drink anything because they were worried that the surgical site could get contaminated and cause a massive infection. I knew they were right, but it didn't make it any easier to endure. My mom came to visit, and I was distant and aloof. She sat in silence next to me, trying to absorb my pain, but we both knew nothing would make the misery less.

There were days of deep loneliness in between my parents' visits. As I lay in the hospital bed, recovering, my restless mind turned toward the future, and I began to start planning and preparing for the reality that was to come. I acknowledged to myself that right now I was in limbo, in a survival state of pain and suffering. But this would eventually end and transition into what would be real life. In many ways, I knew that what I was enduring right now was easier to handle than what lay in the future. The shock of being paralyzed had still not fully worn off, and my survival instinct pushed my body forward day after day. However, the rational part of my brain realized that this would not always be the case, and that once I came home from the hospital, life would be much more difficult. I would have to reinvent myself, and relearn how to live, and how to enjoy my life.

    I tried to set myself up for success and be prepared for what was to come. My mind wandered toward the idea of coming home, and all of the hardships that came with it, both mental and physical. I knew that there would be nothing I could do to avoid it, but mentally preparing for it seemed like it would give me an edge and a better understanding of it when it happened. The suffering I'd already gone through was tremendous, and I knew that eventually there would be a point in my recovery that I could see a future for myself, a future with a full life. I clung to that vision and thought of what my future self would want me to do in the time that I had between now and then. My very practical and pragmatic mind went straight to work looking for the path to success. I knew that the steps would be small, and seemingly inconsequential now. But just like investing money, I knew investing time and effort now would pay off in my future life. I decided then and there that after I recovered, I would take steps each day to push myself, to push myself until it hurt and slowly gain ground either emotionally or physically. These thoughts and plans bounced back and forth around in my brain, helping me to make use of every second to set myself up for success.

Oftentimes when we experience pain or trauma, we feel very isolated, and think that no one could possibly understand what we're going through. However, even if the individual circumstances might change, we have all experienced pain. We are not alone. It is how we recover that makes all the difference. Sometimes we feel that no matter what we do, we cannot get rid of the hurt and pain. But what we can do is offer it up and push ourselves to make the most of our actions, even if our heart is not in it. If we accept that we are feeling miserable, but force ourselves to live, then, eventually, we will be able to overtake our mind and subdue it back to reality. Now, I am not saying that making good life decisions after a tragedy will fix everything, but it will give us the best chance. We are so tempted to numb the pain by turning to something outside of us, often something abusive, like overeating, alcohol, pill addiction, or any other number of destructive habits. The problem with these "remedies" is that they still don't help. We still wake up to the same depressing reality that we had the day before. However, when our minds start to let go of that tragedy and move forward, if we have turned to addictions, those habits stay with us, and we have to battle those demons in addition to everything else. How much better if we had decided to make good decisions early on, constantly pushing ourselves to do things that we knew were good for us. When our minds finally snap out of it, we will have acquired a strong foundation of habits and lifestyle that we have fostered, helping to keep us moving forward and giving us hope. So, embrace the suck, and make the right decisions, because your future self will appreciate it. Additionally, nothing we do will make the pain go away, the pain will always stay with us, like a scar, but we must continue living despite it. And pray. Pray for the strength to persevere. Because we do not have the strength on our own, but only with the grace of God.

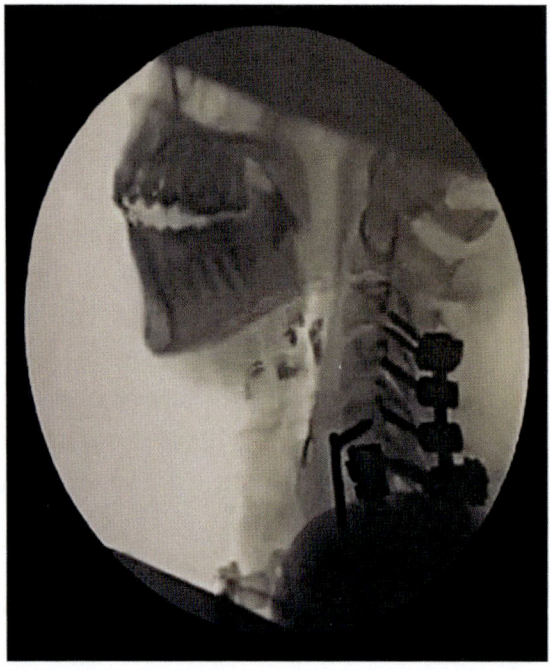

My mom took a picture of the X-ray video watching me swallow. We could not have known that that metal bar holding my spine together had punctured the back of my throat.

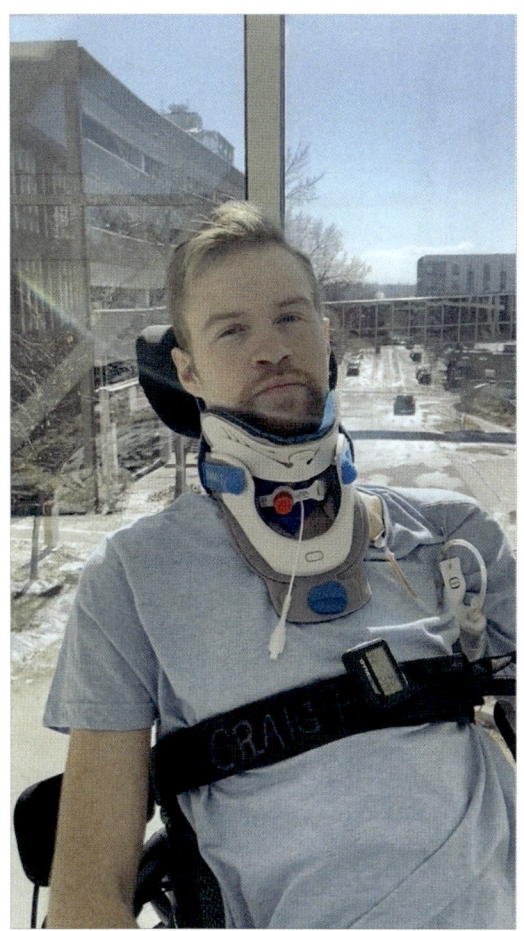

After being told I could not eat and the world felt like it had collapsed around me.

CHAPTER 9

VICTORY!

And then came the day we had been waiting for. The nurse and doctor came in with smiles on their faces and a lightness in their step. They proudly announced that my throat was healed up enough to begin very slowly reintroducing water and mushy foods into my nonexistent diet. I was ready, I thought to myself. I knew I would have to fight the battle of swallowing all over again, but I was resolved to do it, and I was excited to put myself to the challenge. I told my mom to pass on the news to friends and family, and request snack foods of every sort. Boxes and boxes came in, filled with so many delightful treats. It gave me more courage and strength to continue fighting for the ability to eat again. The generosity of so many people was overwhelming. Still to this day, I couldn't be more thankful for what so many people have done for me. I have no doubt that their contributions and prayers have made all the difference in my recovery and continue to give me strength and hope, even now.

    I doubled down my efforts, and my body slowly began to respond, the muscles gradually learned how to operate and remembered their motion. The body felt like it had a mind of its own, but thankfully, in what seemed like the first time since relearning how to breathe, it responded positively. The therapist worked with me during mealtimes to help practice safe swallowing and build up the muscles in my throat. My diet was restricted while my throat healed but just knowing that I was making progress made a huge difference. Each day was filled with different battles, some weighed upon my mind, while others weighed upon my body. I can't say which one was more difficult, only that they each carried with them different challenges and continued to barrage me like a punching bag. The days blended together as I did everything I could to hold on as my body slowly learned to adapt. It was hard, it only took the slightest unexpected failure to tip the scales, and everything came crumbling down. This could be anything from dropping my toothbrush to needing help opening a package. So many hurdles, the gravity of the situation settled in on me, like a dark cloud, covering the landscape in darkness, and making it hard to see what was on the horizon. I prayed at night for the strength to persevere through this darkness, asking our Lord to make the most of my suffering, while I begrudgingly endured what he put in front of me.

Meanwhile my throat was healing up, and my diet slowly shifted from pureed foods to soft foods. This was a huge improvement, given that the pureed foods looked and smelled like dog food and were severely lacking in the taste department. Soft foods were another battle, but at least they tasted better and had the proper consistency for what they were. it felt good to be making progress even if it wasn't as fast as I liked. It was during this time of my recovery that my dad, overexcited about the prospects of me eating and having himself sampled many of the local restaurants, decided to bring some home to me. The foods he brought were definitely not allowed on my diet, but after a little bit of modification it was close enough that I didn't even care. The tastes and the smells were amazing, reawakening sensations and feelings for food that I'd only dreamed of for so long. These little secret meals were like little oases in the desert of recovery, providing me a sample of what life would look like after rehab, and the future that was waiting for me.

It was about a week later that my speech therapist told me they wanted to do another swallow test to determine the results of the surgery and to find out if I was successfully swallowing. Just the thought of going down into the deep, dark dungeon of the radiology department and undergoing that test again filled my mind with so much dread (the devil making every attempt to convince me that I couldn't do it) and despair. I prayed for strength, and then mentally went through all of the steps of the test in my head, visualizing how to go about taking on each different food and beverage, making sure to take a break in between so that I was prepared for the next bite or sip. Finally, I was called down, and after donning the heavy twenty-pound apron and the x-ray was turned on, the test began. It consisted of three levels: the first was a cracker, although in the darkness it looked more like a piece of cardboard, but I knew what was coming for me and made sure to chew it completely so that I could use my saliva to turn it into one giant bolus and swallow it whole. I paced myself and then swallowed hard, willing myself with every ounce of my being to get it down successfully. It felt good, finally my body seemed like it was communicating properly. Next was the pudding. The trick with this one was making sure that it was all toward the back of my throat before I swallowed so that there was no trail left behind that could drip down the wrong pipe. Once again, I took my time, thought it through, and swallowed hard. Nothing felt like it was lingering in the back of my throat. I swallowed again just to make sure and then moved on to the combination of pudding and cracker together. The routine for this one was the same; put it all together in the back of the throat and swallow hard twice. Again, nothing felt wrong. The final test was the hardest—liquids. The reason why liquids were so difficult is that they disperse everywhere, so they could easily spread down into the lungs. I braced myself, trying to pull together every nerve fiber I could to pass the last test. It started with a straw, which was a little easier, because it was a closed system so my body could create one continuous vacuum. Thankfully it went straight down without a problem. Finally, they had me drink straight from the cup, which was more difficult because the liquid spread out, splashing around the inside of my mouth and threatening to sneak down into my lungs. I did everything I could to keep my throat closed until everything was in, and then just like before, I put it all toward the back of my mouth and swallowed hard twice, trying to make sure that nothing was left in my throat that could drip down into my lungs. No coughing or crying, always a good sign. They turned off the x-ray machine and took off the vest, telling me to go back to my room, and wait. It was very anticlimactic and stressful, not knowing where I stood. I had a good feeling but nowhere near enough to feel confident. I went back into my room and waited for the verdict.

    A couple of hours later my doctor and therapist came into the room. The tension was palpable as I waited for them to talk, my mind racing to try to pick up on their body language and facial expressions for any hint of the outcome. As soon as the speech therapist opened her mouth, I knew even before the words came out that I had passed. I did my best to stay calm as I waited for the complete diagnosis, but inside I was bursting with joy. The future suddenly seemed brighter, and another major hurdle had been overcome. They explained to me that not only did I pass with flying colors, but also the surgery looked very successful, and completely healed. Cheers of celebration were exuberantly exchanged back and forth, and I could see how much it also meant to them, as they had been with me throughout the whole process, watching so much sorrow and depression come through my life, and now finally a victory. My dad, who was with me at the time, also looked as though a huge weight had been lifted off his shoulders, seeing this as a sign from God that all was not lost, and things would get better.

 The boost of confidence from hearing that I had passed the test resonated throughout my being and finally allowed me to acknowledge not only how far I'd come, but to have some hope that I could live normally again. It felt good to know that my body had learned to swallow. In a spirit of celebration, my dad went out and purchased two huge burgers with fries. It was one of my favorite meals that I had dreamed of for the last three months. My father filmed me as I opened the package. The smell of the food was intoxicating. I could not believe I was going to eat one of my favorite meals.

 But God was not finished with my humility. I went to pick up the burger and immediately realized the uselessness of my fingers. I gritted my teeth and tried to pick up the burger with my awkward palms. I had only started to lift it to my mouth when the burger flipped out of my hands like a live thing and then fell onto the floor. I looked at it for a moment, simply not believing that after so long of dreaming of eating a burger, I could not even hold it in my hands. My father was matter-of-fact and ordered a second burger. When it came, I was determined to eat it in any way that was necessary. We could deal with motor skills later. I hovered over the plate like a beast and took down the burger and fries without even really lifting them off the plate. It wasn't a pretty sight, but boy was it delicious. The following day we ordered another burger, and this time I had my dad shove it into my fingers so that the natural tension would help keep the burger together. This strategy worked out much better and I was able to enjoy the burger with my hands, and while it was a little messy, it was very rewarding.

One of my favorite moments was when my dad was visiting me during a snowstorm. Everything was covered with two feet of snow outside and we watched through the wide windows as the wind and the snow grew worse. We were just about to go down to dinner when we realized how late it was, and that we had missed the dinner service at the cafeteria. My father looked through every food delivery app and even called a few delivery services in the area. But they all told us the same thing. They had all been shut down due to the blizzard. Hungry, I looked on our map and saw that there was a pizza place open three miles away. It was impossible to drive in the storm. Yet my father did not even hesitate for a second. He smiled and told me not to worry as he put on his jacket. I watched in awe as he left to trudge out into the snow to get me a slice of pizza. He walked six miles through two feet of snow in a pair of tennis shoes and jeans. Not only did he make it to the pizza place and pick up a pizza but even stopped on the way back to help an old lady's car out of the snow. When he finally arrived, he was completely drenched from head to toe. However, instead of complaining, he simply made a joke about how he was sorry that the pizza was cold. Of course I thanked him profusely, but I'm sure the magnitude of the task was way more strenuous than he let on. That memory will live forever in my mind as the greatest example of fatherhood, and one of the best pizzas I've ever had.

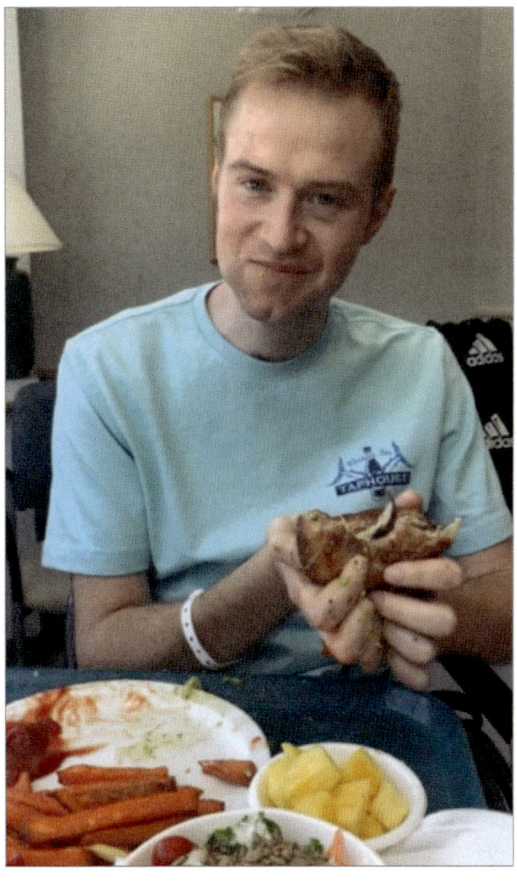

Mastering the hamburger!

CHAPTER 10

AN UNLIKELY ADVENTURE

One day, I told my friend, Chris Waker, who was also paralyzed and in rehabilitation with me, that I wanted us to go on an adventure in the hospital on our own. We decided that the best test of our independence, that was actually a possibility, was to sneak into the break room and try to make tea. It might not sound like a very complicated or difficult task. But when you consider that neither of us had hand function, we were going into a staff break room that was not very wheelchair friendly and trying to pour hot water into a cup, you start to get a better picture of just what we were getting ourselves into.

First, a little bit of context. At this point in my recovery, I still had a lot of excess bone growth in my hips and my spine. It was impossible for me to bend over, so I could not pick anything up off the floor. Additionally, neither of us had core function, so if we bent over, we were unable to pick our upper body up without the use of our arms.

So, with all of these limitations, we pushed our wheelchairs down the hallway. At this point, it was around 9:00 p.m. The hospital was quiet, and nobody was paying too much attention to us. We wheeled into the break room and assessed the situation. There was a hot water dispenser, so that meant this dream was actually a possibility, as we did not have to worry about stoves, or any complicated appliances. The next step was to grab a cup off the counter, which coincidentally was pushed all the way back up against the wall, making it very difficult to reach from a wheelchair. Since I had longer arms, I reached out as far as I could and, with just the tip of my knuckles, was able to knock a Styrofoam cup over toward my body. But I used too much force, and it fell onto the floor. I looked at him, knowing that that cup was our only chance of making the tea, as there were no more cups in reach. He, being the only one with the ability to touch the ground, gave me a look that just said, "Eff it! let's do this!" He bent over to the ground and in his straining and exertion to grab the cup, he crapped his pants. I could barely contain my laughter as he did his best to struggle up to a sitting position by putting the cup in his teeth and bracing his arms to push his body back up. We had retrieved the cup, but we had casualties.

Of course, the next step was to get hot water and tea into the cup, something that we didn't realize was going to be a problem until we got there. I managed to put the cup under the hot water dispenser and filled it up but then was met with the reality of how I was going to get it back to my room, as it was boiling liquid, and I had no table or flat surface to put it on. So, we managed to get a tea bag inside it and mangle a lid on top of it, and then I decided the best thing to do was just to put it between my legs and try to move fast so that it didn't have a chance to burn me through my jeans. We immediately rolled out of the kitchen and headed back to my room. I pushed through the hallways and despite their being flat, managed to bump the hot tea all over myself as I attempted to move quickly.

Thankfully it was no more than drops, and we got back to the room without much further incident. Once I put the cup down on my desk I looked back at Chris and smiled—we had done it! A little glimmer of hope in both our eyes. Despite me burning myself and him crapping his pants, we had managed to make a cup of tea. I knew that adventure would bond us forever, lifelong friends forged through overcoming adversity at all costs. I will always remember that moment, the ability to laugh at our situation, the ability to make light of our misfortunes, and most importantly, the ability to appreciate the little victories amid the suffering. Success never comes without failure, and as long as we keep our end goal in mind, we can deal with the speed bumps along the way and relish the victory we are able to achieve at the end. It felt good to be making friends at Craig Hospital and to be able to laugh at ourselves.

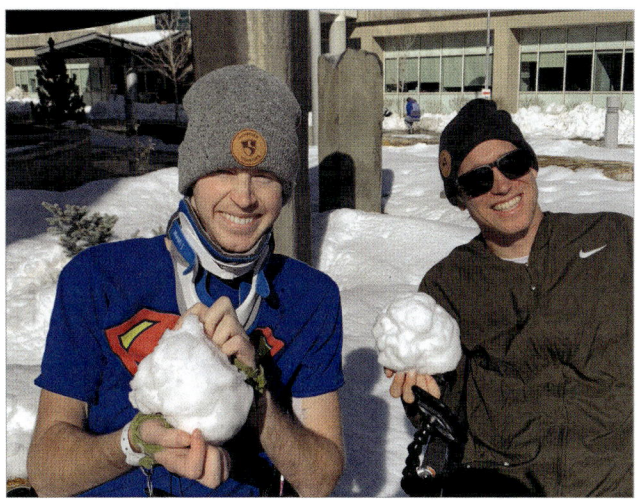

Chris Waker and I having some hilarious form of a snowball fight. We could not feel how cold the snow was on our hands!

CHAPTER 11

PALO ALTO VA

It was not long afterward that I sat down with my social worker for our weekly meeting. I imagined this would be a pretty standard meeting, possibly to discuss the remaining two months of my rehab at Craig Hospital. However, his tone took on some seriousness, as he explained that the military had finally realized that I was on active duty during the accident, and wanted me to come home to California and finish out my rehab at the Palo Alto Veterans Administration (VA). The news was a little surprising, because I had planned on finishing my rehab at Craig Hospital, and yet at the same time it also made sense. I felt sad to be leaving Craig, as I had already grown fond of my nurses and therapists and had made good friends. But after having accomplished so much, I felt prepared to take on the transition and whatever rehabilitation the VA provided.

The day finally arrived for me to leave and my dad began to pack everything. By the time he had finished, I ended up having seventeen boxes of stuff! What a difference from the two duffle bags that I had arrived with. The huge quantity of boxes contained some take-home medical equipment from Craig, but the majority of boxes were filled with the treasured gifts from so many friends, family, and people I didn't even know. There were leftover snacks, Christmas presents, pictures, letters, rosaries, and pictures of saints. So many gifts that helped me to focus on the good to be hoped for, and the good that I still had. Each and every item carried with it a story of someone's love, time, and money that went into showing how much they cared for and were thinking of me. Even complete strangers that I had never met had sent me heartfelt letters and countless prayers. A stream of emotions washed over me as I watched the items being packed away, reliving the moment when I received them and remembering how much love and prayers I had received during my recovery. It was almost overwhelming, seeing it all laid out. I took a moment to thank God for so many people that I could never repay, and how much they'd given me in this time of darkness.

As the boxes got packed up into a shipping truck, I moved on to another difficult task—saying goodbye to the doctors, nurses, therapists, and fellow patients that I'd met. All the people that had seen me at my lowest, and had helped build me up and given me the courage to see a brighter future and make the most of whatever life had in store. I wheeled around the hospital, giving out hugs, and occasionally shedding a tear, telling everyone how much they had meant to me, and knowing that I may never see them again. After all the goodbyes were said, I headed back to my room, where I waited for an ambulance to pick me up and take me to the airport.

The ride to the airport was brief and went by without too much trouble. Unfortunately, due to my fragility and the size of the airplane, they had to carry me lying down. The bed was uncomfortable, but there was nothing to do except lie there and wait. While it seems like everyone's dream is to lie down on an airplane and just sleep until the ride is over, it was anything but for me. The ceiling was only half a foot from my face, my body felt misaligned, and there was phlegm deep down in my lungs that I knew I did not have the strength to cough up. None of these things could be easily fixed or were life-threatening, so I sucked it up and endured the flight, constantly listening for a sign that we were almost there. Thankfully the flight was only a couple of hours, so my suffering was short-lived. We landed in California and took yet another ambulance to my new rehabilitation center at the Palo Alto VA.

I was excited to be back in California, excited as they pulled me out of the ambulance, to see trees and grass. Excited for the warmth of the sun and the warm days ahead. Excited to be closer to my family and friends. I was hopeful for this next step in my recovery, but I was nervous about all of the changes. I didn't know what the new doctors, nurses, or therapists would be like, and prayed that they would be able to help me just as much as the ones at Craig. At Craig Hospital they had all become part of my family, so it was hard to wrap my head around getting used to a whole new support staff.

Once I'd been situated in my new hospital bed, I got to see the lineup of my new medical team. All of the new interactions were difficult for me to keep up with, so many new faces and names that I knew I would immediately forget. I was also drastically aware of how many nurses were foreign and seemed to have limited English. Further, their accents made it hard to understand what they were saying and made communication even harder. Having conversations and asking for things took especially long and was very tedious. I knew they meant well, but in my fragile state it was still all overwhelming. Meanwhile, the Covid restrictions were still in full effect, and so my own family could only visit me through a window. Once again, I felt abandoned and alone. I didn't know where I was, or the people that were taking care of me.

When the first meal came, I thought I would finally find some relief, some comfort in such a cold, isolated space. However, the food was some of the worst I've ever tasted. The main dish was three meatballs soaked with condensation from sitting in a warmer all day, and what looked like canned vegetables and some very questionable gravy. Thankfully, since I was in a big city, there was food delivery, and I immediately made the decision in my head that I would spend the money I needed in order to make sure that I had a warm, filling meal every night. It was a small consolation, but I knew it would help keep me sane during my final months of rehab and help provide me with just a little bit of comfort, and something to look forward to at the end of each day.

After the food, one of the most noticeable differences between the rehabilitation centers was the age gap between me and all of the other spinal cord patients at the hospital. The youngest person I found during my stay was probably thirty years older than me. This made my rehab even harder, as I had no one to commiserate with, no one to rally behind, no one to help keep pushing me forward. There was a lack of companionship, and it took its toll on me. It was hard enough having my life stripped before my eyes, everything I knew flipped on its head, and yet harder still without having anyone else to work through it with. The saying that misery loves company rang over and over again in the back of my head, as I tried to find the strength to push myself alone.

I thought of our Lord, wandering in the desert for forty days and forty nights, thinking about how difficult it must have been to suffer alone, finding the strength to persevere, and resist the temptations of the devil without the companionship of his apostles.

Then Jesus was led by the Spirit into the wilderness to be tempted by the devil. After fasting forty days and forty nights, he was hungry. The tempter came to him and said, "If you are the Son of God, tell these stones to become bread." Jesus answered, "It is written: Man shall not live on bread alone, but on every word that comes from the mouth of God" (Matthew 4:1).

I took comfort in knowing that what I had to endure God had endured before me, and would be with me through it all. I had only to trust in him and keep pushing forward, no matter how rocky the road would be.

Upon getting to Palo Alto, it seemed like no one was in a rush to get started. Instead of having physical therapy and occupational therapy every day, I felt more like I was having it once a week. I missed how organized and complete the schedule at Craig Hospital was. This lack of consistency was bad for both my morale and my drive. I was begging to get stronger, to learn more, to adapt, and learn how to overcome the obstacles that I knew would come my way. However, due to the way their system was set up and the type of patients they had, this was not something they were used to, and not something they had the resources to fulfill. Therefore, I made sure to make the most of the visits I did have. I had learned enough from Craig Hospital that I could help train myself when I wasn't with them.

The weeks passed slowly, my entertainment consisted of binge-watching TV shows and talking with friends and family when they came to visit outside my window. Visiting was difficult but everybody made it work and brought many gifts, consisting mostly of snacks and fresh fruit, commodities that were very difficult for me to get at the hospital. I enjoyed having visitors, but at the same time, seeing so many of my old friends made my accident that much more real. The juxtaposition of where I was with seeing them continuing to live their lives, sent pangs of sorrow down to the very depths of my core. The nagging thoughts of just how unfair it seemed began to gnaw at me. I did my best to keep emotions controlled and continue living the life that God had put in front of me. Instead of being able to fade into the darkness, I had chosen to face my life head-on. It was a hard thing to do, to see your friends and others live the life you wanted to have and realize that it will never be yours. Their visits, while so loving and enjoyable, at the same time cut deep into my heart and for a moment, I was thankful for the window. Thankful for just a little bit of separation that allowed me to emotionally distance myself from reality. I allowed myself to mourn after they had left, thinking of all of the memories I had with friends and family from activities, interactions, and times gone by. So many little details flooded into my mind like torture, not letting me find any peace, but instead drawing attention to every inadequacy and disability I had. The rational part of my brain kept saying "Wait, be patient, time will help heal these moments, new memories will form, and you will have a new life." But the emotional part of my brain wouldn't give me any peace. It made me sad and depressed. I was unable to shake the feeling that what I lost would forever inhibit my ability to relate to these people again. I felt like I was a mere shadow of the man that I used to be. I felt unable to find consolation in my situation and felt constantly reminded of my terrible loss.

While I know there are a lot of difficult things that come with a traumatic injury, I also know that this feeling is one shared by many. I do not pretend to know exactly how to speak to everyone's situation, but I do know that such a trauma hits hard, leaving a dark tunnel with seemingly no way out. And while time helps heal all wounds, we must always remember that from the first moment of our trauma, God is with us. He is a light by our side even in our darkest moments. Even when we are in pain, feel lost, and do not know the way, he is always there. He sees our suffering and is asking for us to unite it to him on the cross. There we join him and make a sacrifice for our soul and the salvation of many others. It is through this offering that we learn to love God above ourselves and grow every day in perfect glorification of him.

When I first arrived at the VA, a nurse told me, "This will be your new home away from home." After the luxury of Craig Hospital, this seemed like a comment from a horror movie. But after a few weeks there, I began to get to know the nurses and especially my doctor, Dr. Kim. They all tried so hard to help me, to listen to me, and to explain things to me. Dr. Kim soon realized I had some medical knowledge from my schooling and so she took the time to explain medical procedures, or problems. I'm pretty sure she put it in my notes, as other doctors also took the time to explain things. This gave me some small feeling of being in control of my medical state and journey and also really helped me when I went home.

As therapy continued, and I got further in my recovery, one of the topics that came up was nerve transfer surgery for my hands. Due to my injury I had no ability to move my fingers. Even the most simple tasks were ten times more difficult because I could not pick things up with any confidence. Nerve transfer surgery would help bring some of the function back to my hands, not completely but it would allow me to get just a little bit more functionality. The plan was to have one surgery now and another a year or two later. The first surgery involved detaching nerves in my arm from one muscle group and reattaching them to another muscle group that was still functioning. So while some strength would decrease from my forearm muscles, I would get an increase in finger function. While this technique has had many successful operations, it was still not a sure thing. With maybe only 85 percent of people having successful function afterward. Even if the surgery was successful, at best I would only get a small amount of functionality back in my hands.

These hands that had done so much for me in the past. These hands that God had made and imbued with natural talents, allowing me to be the top of my class in dental school and create beautiful works of art out of simple blocks of wood. My hands that had toiled in the field, working to build fences and dig ditches. My hands that had built calluses and scars from many adventures and hard work. My hands that had given me the ability to high-five, shake, salute, and pray the rosary. Oh, how I wished they could just sew all the nerves back together and that my hands could work like they did before. It was hard knowing that would never happen, and I offered it up to God. I stared down at my hands, lifeless, unmoving, and cold; unable to obey my mind's simplest request, seemingly dead yet still attached to me. I knew that even the smallest amount of function given back to my hands would make a huge difference not only for the function, but also the mental shift of realizing that they still had purpose in them. I knew that the surgery was not a perfect solution, but it was the only one available to me, and I was willing to take the risks and deal with all of the recovery needed to get something back. I talked through the pros and cons and finally decided to go for it, trusting that prayer and the Holy Spirit had guided me into making a good decision.

The recovery process was pretty brutal, because they were doing both hands at the same time, so I had to have both of them splinted for a month. During the recovery, I was unable to feed myself or complete a lot of basic daily tasks—something I had fought so hard for in the last several months. It was absolutely humbling to, once again, be so reliant on other people, especially since I had finally gotten some independence. Things like brushing my teeth, combing my hair, or even using my phone were at the mercy of others. Requiring so much assistance immediately triggered my PTSD of the early dark days in the ICU, and there was an immediate attitude change. I struggled drastically to find happiness during that time. Watching TV and videos got boring very quickly, and my only real consolation and outlet for my frustration was prayer and contemplation. It helped me to pray, and listen to Mass, while letting the Holy Spirit guide my thoughts regarding the future of my suffering.

Suffering is horrible, it is also hard to understand why our bodies and minds are so temperamental, fluctuating from happiness one second to utter devastation the next, all the while, not being able to control it. What possible good can it do? An analogy that has always helped me understand suffering, at least from a practical human perspective, is thinking of it like investing money.

We are told that suffering leads to a greater good, but we don't always know what that good is. When someone asks us why we have faith that our suffering is leading to a greater good, all we can do is point to the good that has come from Christ's suffering or the suffering of the saints. In the same way, we know that investing our money is a good thing and leads to even greater rewards. While we know this is true, we often have no idea where our money is going and how it's multiplying. Furthermore, when someone asks us why we are investing, and what our money is doing, we have a hard time explaining the details. Even if we have seen the success and financial gains of others who have invested.

So, while we might not always see the big picture, or know exactly how our lives are affecting other people, we must have faith that our suffering is an investment for our souls and the souls of others. An investment in which the stocks always go up, and our fruits are always multiplied. "And everyone who has left houses or brothers or sisters or father or mother or children or fields, for my name's sake, will receive a hundredfold, and will inherit eternal life" (Matthew 19:29).

Suffering is investing for retirement. Every time we invest, we feel like we are losing out on money we could spend right now, but we do it anyway because we know that by offering it up, we will be rewarded that much more in the future. In addition, we make dividends on what we invest while we are still alive, in the form of diverse blessings and perspectives that God gives us from our suffering. So, while I feel like I do not have as much to spend right now, you better bet everything I save is going to go toward a big retirement party in heaven.

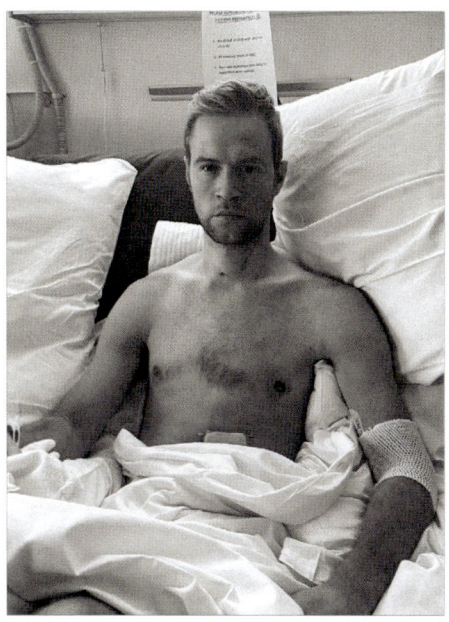

My first day at the Palo Alto VA. I was angry and depressed.

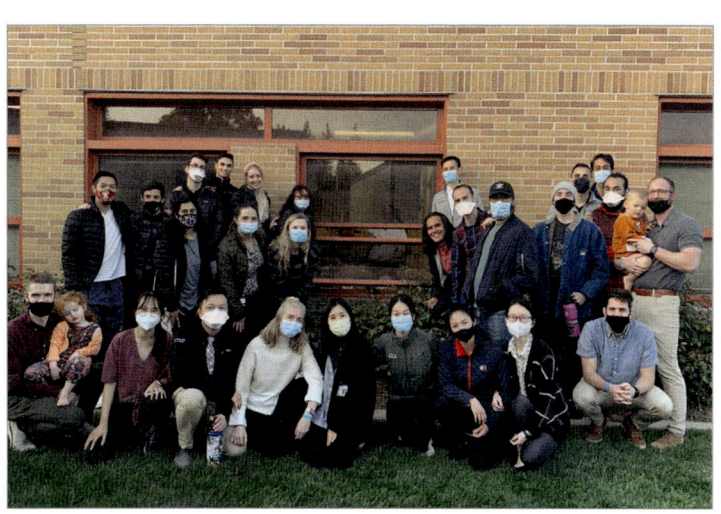

My dental class visiting me outside the window.

CHAPTER 12

MARIPOSA STRONG AND HOME

After a month of recovery, the bandages finally came off, and I was able to use my arms again. A huge sigh of relief, and motivation to get stronger and keep pushing forward. It was the last step of rehab before I was allowed to go home. After so many surgeries, and so many months of rehab, I was excited and terrified to come home. I knew it would be a huge blessing and relief to be around my family again, but I also knew that home would never look the same; there were so many reminders of things that used to be, so many people that I interacted with and would never be able to interact with in the same way again. So many memories were now like nightmares as they only served to freshen the wound that much more. I loved my family, but even the thought of interacting with them pierced my heart. I prayed "Lord, please give me the strength, for I do not have what it takes on my own, but with your grace I can manage."

We made the long drive to Mariposa. Home. I was overwhelmed as we passed the county line and suddenly lights and sirens went off in front of us. The local sheriff had organized a police escort. I was humbled and tears of gratitude formed in my eyes. As we came closer to our house, I saw banners on the road, banners and people, waving for miles to celebrate my return. I could not form words. I did not deserve it. Their love was overwhelming. It helped me to realize that others cared about me, and that God cared about me even more. I was beyond thankful for the support from my community and my friends. This gave me confidence as I began my recovery, knowing that they would help me every step of the way. I knew I was not alone, and that with the help of others I would succeed. We have a saying in Mariposa: "Mariposa Strong." It has been used over and over to encourage each other in times of hardship—fire that devastated 80 percent of the community, a sheriff hurt badly in the line of duty, another fire that took the life of a firefighter, floods that took down bridges and took lives with them. In all these times of sorrow and hardship, our community has come together to support and encourage each other. Our little town is blessed with its courage and strength. We have always tried to do what we could to help and I was touched to the core to be on the receiving end of such love and support.

Support was definitely needed, as the return home was much more difficult than I could ever have anticipated. The memories came flooding back immediately. So many things were different, so many sights and sounds brought to mind such deep memories in my brain. Memories that carried so much sorrow, as they felt so hollow now. My mind began to play out those memories in my head. Our ranch had been such a playground for me and my brothers and sisters. We had built roads for the horses and tough terrain vehicles. We had built forts, patios, swimming holes and jumps. I could no longer get out to the back of the property as my wheelchair could not navigate the rough terrain and even if I could, I could not bear to see the place of so much fun, creativity, and hard work. I could not bear to see the swimming hole where we jumped in at the first blush of cold spring sunlight. I could not bear to see the jump we made by burying old tires and the back of an old van seat. I could not bear to see the long winding fence we put in with my family when we first moved and dreamed of all the animals it would hold. All this was lost to me now, and the pain was suffocating.

I quickly shut the door and didn't allow my mind to progress further down the rabbit hole. I shut my mind off and forced it to stay in the present, forced it to live for the next moment, and the one after that, preventing it from diving into a tailspin of sorrow for all that was lost. I knew that I could only hold the floodgates back for so long before everything would eventually burst through, but I knew that I must focus on the task at hand and get through the day.

My little brothers, whom I spent so many hours teaching how to dig holes and build fences, now happily offered to be my caregivers, relieving the physical task from my mom and the searing heartbreak from my dad. I had taught my little brothers how to have a strong work ethic and how to make workout programs to get strong. Little did we know, it would be used to help me get out of bed or take a shower. It was terribly humbling, but I was also so proud of them. Those two boys, who were goofy, fun loving, and had hearts of gold, did not think twice about devoting an hour in the morning before school and an hour at night to help me.

My parents and a family friend who did construction worked like crazy to rebuild my bedroom to adapt to my new needs. My four brothers and I had always shared a bedroom. It was very small, much like the size of a large closet and it was a crazy mess of toys and clothes with paintball guns and bows and arrows hanging on the wall. We had painted it ourselves, a dark army green. When I came home, it was a clean blue and gray, with an attached bathroom. My parents were so proud to show it to me. It was beautiful and perfect, but I missed the crazy mess that I needed to jump over just to leap into bed. That perfectly tiled floor was for someone in a wheelchair.

Being home was full of constant reminders of my limitations, like needing to ask for help to move toys or random things in my way as I tried to maneuver throughout the house. Or needing to ask someone to get me food when I was hungry. These constant little, yet annoying, tasks wore on me, making it difficult to not feel like a burden and that I was living in a world where I didn't belong.

It was very hard going from being independent, capable, and successful, to being so utterly dependent on others, and to struggle with every little thing. I believe many people don't understand the extreme complexity of what comes with a spinal cord injury. Most people just assume that someone in a wheelchair is just someone that cannot walk. They brush it off and then don't give it a second thought. But the reality is much more dramatic than that. Not being able to walk is just the tip of the iceberg. Spinal injuries cause nerve damage, which results in extreme nerve pain throughout the body where there is otherwise no sensation. There is often little or no feeling below the level of injury, making it difficult to keep track of potential damage to the skin and tissues because you cannot feel it. There is no muscle innervation below the level of injury, which can be misleading because a lot of people just assume it's at the hips, but oftentimes it can mean no use of the fingers, no control or strength in the core, no back muscle, and no triceps, making even the simplest of tasks dramatically more complicated.

There are also bladder and bowel difficulties, as there is no longer the same control as before, so in order to drain urine, a catheter must be used, either an indwelling catheter or intermittently cathing every time the bladder needs to be emptied. For bowel stimulation a suppository is needed to trigger an automated response from the body to empty fecal matter, commonly referred to as a bowel program, which can take several hours. There is poor circulation throughout the body, resulting in much lower energy, and difficulty regulating temperature. Even though sex is still possible, there is decreased coordination between the sympathetic and parasympathetic nervous systems, making it much more difficult to have children naturally. Almost all spinal cord injuries result in the body's inability to sweat, causing thermal regulation to be a serious and even life-threatening issue if not managed properly. The body in its weakened state and without support of muscles is also more prone to respiratory diseases, blood clots, and many other secondary conditions that can be life-threatening. This list doesn't do justice to the wide plethora of difficulties that come along with a spinal cord injury.

I had a constant battle in my soul between accepting things the way they were and struggling to move on to something greater. Even worse, I refused to give myself credit for any of my accomplishments. I dismissed them as insignificant, and I flat out rejected praise from my family. It felt meaningless and almost cruel to be praised for tasks that were so small and which it seemed like anyone could do. I constantly had to remind my family not to treat me differently or pamper me. This made my own recovery more difficult. My parents especially did not understand. One time my mom asked for someone to pass the salt. I jokingly grabbed the salt and threw it at her. It almost hit her and then fell to the floor. She picked it up and said, "Nice throw." I immediately got frustrated. Not only was it a terrible throw, but I knew as well as anyone else that throwing was not allowed at the table. I said as much to her and watched her face change from sorrow to anger and at last to understanding.

My only relief came from pushing myself. Each day I challenged myself to tackle something new, regardless of how small. Sometimes the successes were major, and I was able to achieve things that I was proud of, and other days it was a basic necessity of life, like brushing my teeth or getting my own coffee. I continued to work out and rejoiced that I was able to get stronger. This attitude always gave me something to fight for each day and gave me the ability to see past the pain and achieve something greater.

But our Lord also gave me small blessings, especially with my little nephew. He kept me smiling as he asked for wheelchair rides and to go around the house looking for bugs. I enjoyed his companionship, knowing that he did not view me in any way differently, nor did he have any expectations of conversation or intellectual thought, but merely just enjoyed spending time with me, or maybe enjoyed me as a practical mode of transportation to his next adventure. It did me good to watch him live and helped me step away from my worries for a second. I could bring joy and happiness to him without any fear of disappointment or worry about inadequacy. It was a small view into how our Lord sees our little acts of kindness and prayer. He, above everyone else, appreciates our small sacrifices, and they never go unnoticed. Never consider anything we do for our Lord to be too small; he accepts all of these offerings and appreciates them more than anyone else ever could.

I decided to try 3-D printing, creating the images on the computer and then giving the command to the printer. I had a lot of fun making toys for my nieces and nephews, as well as a Settlers of Catan 3-D board set which we all painted as a Christmas project. I also began to set myself up for a job in the near future. As long as my brain and body were being pushed and challenged, I was able to stave off the giant cloud of depression that was trying to catch up to me. Although I knew this was only a temporary solution, it helped me get through a lot of the worst parts of my recovery. The moments that I couldn't avoid, I prayed and offered up to God, knowing that as long as I was doing his will, he would take care of the rest.

But he is a faithful God, always at my side, helping me and giving me the daily grace to push forward. As summer progressed, I started to fall into a routine. I woke up at 9:30 a.m. to take care of my personal hygiene, have breakfast, work out, and then spend time on hobbies. The length to which I successfully completed each of these things depended drastically on my energy level. I tried hard not to get frustrated as I fought against my body, making sure to set myself up for success by gradually adding more things into my life when I could handle them. Working out was especially difficult. Before my accident, exercising had come easily without a second thought, and now even picking up the weights was a challenge. Half of my muscles didn't work, the other half were weak, and on top of that I had no strength in my core, and so I had no ability to balance. Every movement took so much coordination and willpower to complete, my energy was taxed just setting up to do an exercise, let alone actually accomplishing it. I tried to drown out my overthinking with music and just keep pushing. It was a hard task, but I closed my eyes, acknowledged my limitations, and just lifted the damn weights. Each day was a struggle, but with each hurdle I overcame there was a glimmer of hope.

Fall came and the days grew shorter and cooler. The boys went back to school, and I was left alone. I tried to stay busy, but in the quiet times, I noticed my mom was worried. And then I overheard her talking to my dad about my brothers' schooling. She had been called by the school telling her they had missed too many days of school, showed up late for too many classes, and were in danger of failing out. This wore heavy on my heart. I prayed about it and talked to my brother Bernhard who was newly married and working at a very good job. He offered to leave his job and be my caretaker. My parents were in the process of building a new home and he suggested living in our old home, right next door. I was moved by his generosity, and also glad to have a more permanent caretaker since I knew the boys would soon be off at college and definitely not able to help. I was also glad for Bernhard's personality. He is quick tempered, quick with a joke, wholly indifferent to emotions and very smart. He had also been trained as an EMT. He would be a perfect companion to not let me feel sorry for myself, the perfect companion to challenge me to independence, and smart enough to help with some of the complexities of my medical care. And so, as the boys returned to school in earnest, Bernhard and his wife and new little son settled in next door and Bernhard began as my caretaker. It has been a good relationship over the past three years. We have had both laughs and trials as well as plenty of emergencies, but his care has been pivotal in my recovery.

I started being able to take over some basic necessities in life, and developed a routine that I could do independently. This helped me to grow in mental fortitude, and the endorphins raced back in as I started making progress. As long as I realized that I was running my own race and forgot about comparing myself to everyone else, I was succeeding. However, because there was no one else to fight against except myself, I knew I was in for some stiff competition. Any measure of success that I found was by pushing myself past my limits. The old adage of the turtle and the hare took on a whole new meaning as I began to realize that judging my success by comparison to others was shallow and didn't fully push me to become my best. Nevertheless, it was hard to keep that in mind when the entire world judged success by comparison between people. However, it is only the Lord that knows the heart and the talents that he has given to each of us. Therefore, let us strive to always be the best we can be regardless of how we compare to others, either higher or lower. Let us never become complacent or slow down lest we fall behind in God's eyes and fail to finish the race.

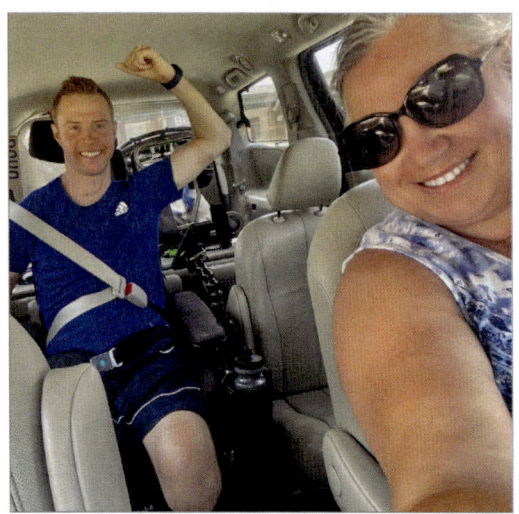

Driving home to Mariposa and seeing the Mariposa Sheriffs escorting me when we crossed the county line. It felt so good to be coming home!

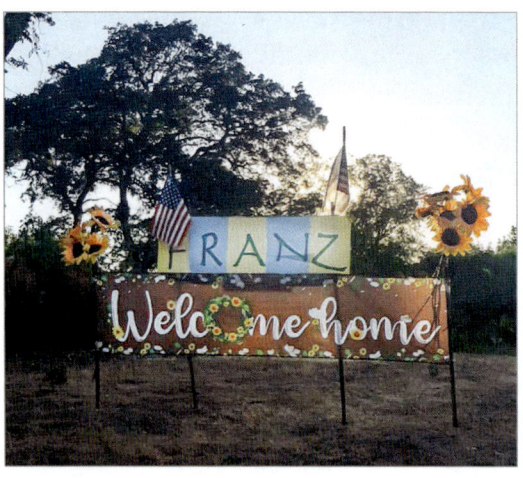

The community posted signs all along my route home, welcoming me and encouraging me. It meant so much to me to have their support!

CHAPTER 13

THE CYST

Just as I was starting to get used to my routine and felt like I was finally getting stronger, something changed. It started off faint, and barely noticeable, but my right arm was starting to slowly get more numb, and my muscles were getting weaker instead of stronger. It was strange, and I didn't understand what was happening. Recalling my years of experience from working in the gym, I thought maybe I was just sore, and my muscles were weak. I decided to take a couple of rest days in the hopes that I would soon be back to normal and ready to work out again. But the truth was much scarier than I could have ever imagined. As my symptoms were quickly getting worse, and not only worse, but dramatically worse, I began to panic. I called the doctor and let them know what was going on, expressing my sense of urgency and concern. They listened to everything I had to say and recommended that I get an MRI and send them the results.

The following day I went straight to the emergency room. The doctor ordered an MRI on my brain and spinal cord to help understand what was happening and determine how serious it was. I thought about looking up what it could be, except with little to go on, I knew that Web MD would turn up with so many misleading results that I was more likely to receive a diagnosis of pregnancy than anything helpful. I decided to wait.

I sat there in the emergency room. It must have been a strange morning because I was surrounded by people who were screaming, wincing, and in agonizing pain. Forced to sit and witness so much suffering, I was drawn to the reality of hell and eternal suffering. "In that place there shall be wailing and gnashing of teeth" (Matthew 13:48).

I know that hell is very real, and along with it is eternal suffering. What little pain we experience on this earth is nothing compared to eternity. While this knowledge doesn't make the suffering any easier, it does help put it into perspective. The suffering in hell is eternal and produces no good. However, on earth, we can join our suffering to Christ and share in the salvation of souls, both our own and others. So when you suffer, do not lose hope. We are each given different suffering to offer up. We are all warriors and each of us needs to rally behind the cross and push forward. We only have one life, and we must not waste it wallowing in our suffering, but courageously march forward, bearing it well. And so it goes, that God so often gives us the antidote before the problem. How much I would dwell on this very wisdom in the days and months that followed.

My thoughts were interrupted by the nurse calling me back into the room to take the MRI, which went by without too much difficulty, and the results were immediately sent out to the Palo Alto VA spinal cord unit.

The doctor called me. "It doesn't look good," he said with altogether too much gravity. I held my breath as he explained that there was a growth in my spinal cord, slowly suffocating and blocking off the neurons enervating my arms and my breathing. It was a terrifying moment to realize that what little capability I had was being either further diminished or taken away. The news hit me hard, there was nothing I could do to fix it. I knew no amount of hard work and resilience on my part would affect the outcome. I collected all of the information I could and passed it along to my spinal cord doctor at the Palo Alto VA. They took a look at it and said they needed to call in some specialists to read the MRI results and help diagnose the situation to determine the severity of it.

I had only been home for a couple of months, and already I was headed back to the hospital with a worsening condition. My spirit was crushed, and the thoughts of the future and the grim reality of my situation weighed upon me. I felt like a broken record, going through the same thought process every time. Wasn't getting paralyzed enough? Why must I go through this all over again? As often as I have had these thoughts, somehow it always comes out of nowhere and seems so unfair. I bit my tongue and let our Lord know that I accepted his fate, whatever it may be, even if I didn't understand it. I barely had time to hug my family before taking an ambulance to Palo Alto for more testing.

They ran several more scans and tests, and then the somber news was delivered to me. It was in fact, a cyst, and it was getting bigger at a rapid pace. My heart dropped. There were two treatment options, and unfortunately, both of them were not very likely to be successful. My heart dropped again. Either do surgery to place a drain in the cyst and hope that it would not cause further damage, or they could give me corticosteroids for three weeks to see if they could help bring down the swelling. I asked a bunch of questions about the successfulness of the surgeries, and the likelihood that steroids would help. Most of the answers I got pointed to the fact that unfortunately, the success was not consistent, and there was just not a lot known about the specific situation to be able to give an accurate success rate. I asked for the rest of the day to make a decision. The doctor shook his head and told me I had to hurry with a decision. If surgery was what I desired, it needed to be done soon. The doctor left, and I set my jaw, determined to push the emotions behind me and make a strong analytical decision on what to do next. My mom was with me at the VA and was also in disbelief. We talked it through and decided to start with steroids, because it wasn't permanent, and it was less invasive. If that didn't work, then we could move forward with the surgery.

I went back home and began taking the steroids, and immediately my body started to get catatonic. My face swelled up, I got massive acne, and I scarcely had the strength to move. Every day felt worse than the last, with barely enough energy to eat food every day, spending the rest of the time lying on my back and wishing I was dead. My prayers became more and more desperate, asking our Lord to take me out of my misery, and bring me to him. My spirit was crushed, and I couldn't see a future where my life made sense. All felt lost, and my sense of purpose ended. Everything I had known up to this point, all of my strength and perseverance, had faded, giving rise to desperation and the sad reality of my situation. My spirit and body had been crushed with no relief in sight. Many thoughts ran through my head. The only thing I could do was pray and contemplate, knowing that my suffering was being offered to keep souls out of hell.

The sad reality was that I continued to get worse. It became obvious that the treatment the doctors had prescribed wasn't working, and I was now losing motion and sensation in my other arm. I felt so confused inside, because all I wanted to do was push on and continue to fight. I wanted to get stronger and take on the world. I want to scream out, "Coach, put me in!"

The struggle between my natural instinct and our Lord's will felt so different. However, it was through this that the Lord allowed me to see something profound and yet so easy to take for granted: that it was his will that must be fulfilled, and not my own.

"Take up your cross, deny yourself, and come follow me."

Never have the words "deny yourself" stood out to me so clearly. We must be willing to give up everything in order to be the soldiers that Christ wants us to be. So while my fight might look different from what I thought I was preparing for, I will continue to push on, and I will continue to fight as I know that our Lord will show me the way.

"I am here Lord, I come to do your will."

Contemplating our Lord and his words and sacred scripture gave me some consolation in such a distressing time. Reading his words brought me renewed strength to continue living out his will to the best of my ability.

My life before this accident was filled with so much prestige and success, I had it all—career, brains, physique, and achievement. My life was what many considered perfect. God had graced me in abundance. Then in one instant it was taken away. While I have spent many nights and days lamenting the loss of my former life, it gave me a chance to really reflect on our true purpose on this earth. "If you belonged to the world, the world would love you as its own.

Because you do not belong to the world, but I have chosen you out of the world—therefore the world hates you" (John 15:19). Our sole purpose on this earth is to glorify God: "So whether you eat or drink, or whatever you do, do everything for the glory of God" (1 Corinthians 10:31).

But how can we glorify God on this earth? While the answer to this might be different for each person, I am especially drawn to the words of St. John the Baptist: "I must decrease so that he may increase" (John 3:30). John's willingness to decrease in the eyes of the world took all of the attention off his own accomplishments and turned them back toward Christ. The success and following he had gained in this world, he gave over to Christ and then faded into the background.

I look at my own life and see how so much of my earthly glory has been stripped from me. It seemed like everything I valued was gone in the blink of an eye. But my accomplishments have not disappeared without a purpose, for in decreasing in the eyes of the world, all honor and eminence has been given to God. Any success or achievement that I accomplish now more perfectly reflects God's power, rather than my own, working through me.

So let us not be dismayed if our best efforts seem to fail, our hard work goes unnoticed, we don't stack up to the worldly view of success, or pain and suffering abound. For our purpose in this world is not to bring attention and praise to ourselves, but to reflect the glory of God.

"For thine is the kingdom, and the power, and the glory, forever" (Matthew 6:9).

After three weeks, my body had almost completely shut down, and I was still getting weaker. I looked and felt like I was dying. My family walked with me as best they could, and I knew my parents' hearts were breaking. But this journey was one I had to travel alone. Alone with our Lord who was the best company I could have.

I knew there was only one more chance to improve my current condition and possibly get back a fraction of the strength that I had before the cyst. I talked to the doctor and told him how much of my strength and energy had gone. After a brief conversation, we decided to go ahead with the surgery. The risks of the surgery were great; there was a chance that I could lose proprioception in my body, which meant losing the ability to know where my limbs were in space. This would be extremely disorienting and make it even harder for me to complete my daily tasks. Additionally, because the surgery was on the spinal cord, there was a real danger of causing further damage just trying to drain the cyst. It was a small space and not a lot of room to work, requiring a lot of precision, and any accidental slip could cause permanent damage. Finally, the drain that they were inserting into the cyst was known to plug up, because it was so small. If it became clogged and the cyst grew back, it would require a whole new surgery, a whole new invasive procedure, and another three to six months of recovery. Even if it didn't clog immediately, the catheters only had a lifespan of several years before they clogged anyway. Meaning that going into it, even if everything was successful, I would probably still have to come in three to five years later to do it all over again with the same risks, and the same dangers as before—some even greater than before, due to the developed scar tissue and recurring trauma to the area. And last, but not least, even if the cyst was drained and everything went according to plan, it might not bring back any sensation or strength, but instead might just stabilize me in my current weakened state.

All of these horrors were bouncing around my head during the conversation, but what choice did I have? It was a Catch-22, neither option a clear winner. I had to try and just pray that God would take care of the rest. So, the surgery was scheduled for the following Friday, giving enough time for the steroids to clear my body and give me whatever strength I could muster to handle the surgery. As the reality of the seriousness of this surgery bore down on me, I was inspired to write this prayer, offering up my anxiety and fear of the unknown to our Lord and letting him take care of the outcome.

> Out of the depths I cry to you my God
> Though you feel so far from me, I know you are there
> In my weakness, you are there
> In my suffering, you are there
> In my desolation, you are there
> In my depression, you are there
> In my pain, you are there
> In my unrest, give me peace
> In my confusion, give me peace
> In my loss, give me peace
> In my difficulty understanding your plan, give me peace
> Oh Lord, I know you have not abandoned your humble servant, you are always with me. May you make yourself known to me in this suffering. Allow me to feel your presence in my loneliness. You who know the inner workings of my heart, fill me with the strength to persevere.

The prayer was simple and yet filled me with a profound sense of peace, knowing that I didn't have to worry, whatever the outcome: God was in charge. It would happen just as he intended. Being able to relieve myself of that burden was freeing. I just had to respond to the grace that he gave me to handle the situation. Little did I know that our Lord was giving me the tools to handle what was still to come.

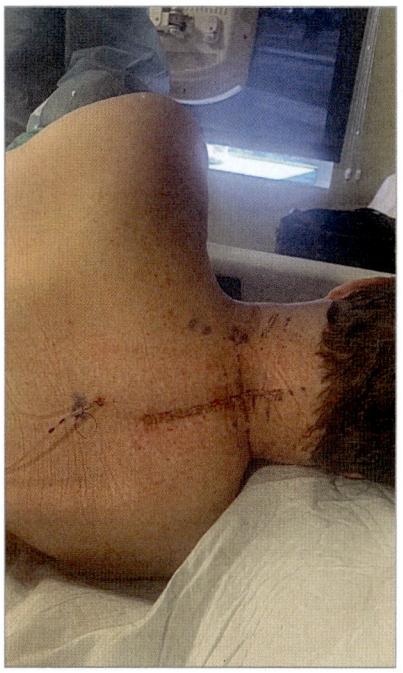

The scar after my cyst surgery

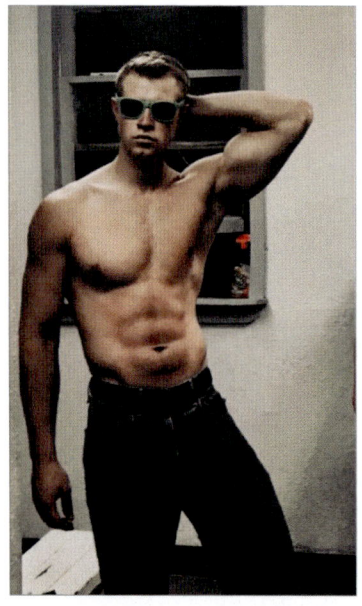

A photo of me at the height of my strength.

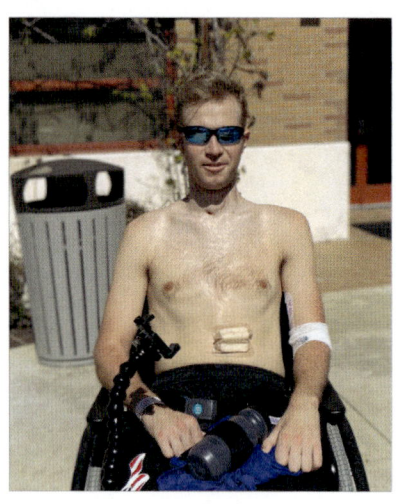

A photo at the end of my stay at the VA, the sum total of destruction on my wasted and paralyzed body.

CHAPTER 14

THROUGH THE DARKNESS

Friday morning came faster than I had anticipated, and before I knew it, I was in the waiting room to prepare for surgery. The neurosurgeon came in and reassured me, telling me that this was the only viable option, and that they would do the best they could to deliver a successful result. The way he phrased it, although reassuring, also struck a chord with how dangerous this operation really was, and there were no guaranteed results. I prayed, asking our Lord to guide the surgeon's hands, hoping for the best, knowing that the next several hours could make all the difference for what the rest of my life would look like. I went through all their standard questions and precautions, and then they wheeled me into the surgery room and put the gas mask on, and I slowly drifted off to sleep.

When I woke up, my head was in a daze, trying to find where I was in this haze of reality. I finally realized that I was still waiting in a hospital bed to be transferred back to the recovery unit. I knew at that moment it was going to be a long and painful recovery. My head ached, my neck was stiff, and I felt terrified to move, knowing that it would hurt more. I closed my eyes, and prayed that sleep would take me, and that recovery would be quick. Unfortunately, that was not the case. I continually woke up with intense pain, begged the nurses for some pain medication, and prayed to God that at least my suffering would be offered up for the salvation of souls.

The next week I wasn't even allowed to lift the head of my bed up for fear that the inflammation would prolong recovery and affect the surgical site. This made it extremely difficult to eat, and when I did eat, it was usually something small and easy to get down so that I did not choke. Thankfully, I was really tired, so the days passed by quickly with a delirious mix of daydreaming and sleeping. My mom came to visit, and I could see the strain and worry on her face. Her pain made mine all the more present, but I couldn't think about that. I had to simply focus on getting better. I had to focus on my own emotional journey and physical recovery, and knew I wasn't able to juggle anything else. My mother understood that, and she suffered silently along with me.

It's so easy to talk about surgery and the horrors of suffering in retrospect, because the words on the page don't completely represent the reality of emotional and physical turmoil. Even now as I write, the words go through my mind and onto the page without my feeling or being able to fully convey the intense pain and suffering from that surgery. In the same way, reading about our Lord's passion and suffering doesn't do justice to the horrible pain that our Lord had to endure for our sake. It doesn't do justice to how much he suffered for our sins, how he knew we would sin again and yet he still offered it up for us. Praying and thinking of our Lord and the great sacrifice he made for us, helped give me the strength to offer up mine in union with him.

Pushing Through the Pain

As my body and mind gradually got stronger, I began to feel the psychological pain of being stationary for so long and being unable to move. Being trapped in bed for so long was very depressing, and it was hard to enjoy any minute of it, let alone the three weeks that I had to spend in acute recovery. When I finally got the all-clear to go into my chair again, the pain was excruciating, and every movement was like a bolt of lightning running down my spine. Everything was baby steps: making it to the chair and spending all day not moving on it, slowly graduating to wheeling around my hospital room, and finally trying to eat by myself. Each setback and difficulty triggered the PTSD I had when I faced the same challenges earlier in my recovery. Each step brought fresh reminders of my condition, and how far I still had to go.

Eventually my pain started to subside, and my energy level started to return. A date was planned for me to return home. However, as much as I was looking forward to going home, I knew much more work and struggle would take place there as well. I knew that things would only improve if I put in the time and work. I kept pushing myself, not allowing myself to look backward. Going home was in fact a challenge, and I struggled mentally, resisting the urge to compare my new weakness with my old strength. I wasn't even thinking of how things were before the accident, I was just taken aback by how difficult they were since the surgery. So many pessimistic thoughts scratched at the back of my mind, begging to be released, begging to take control of my mind and send it into a spiral of depression. I once again fought back the urge to give in, and instead, offered it up to our Lord to make of it what he willed. I tried to drown out the evil thoughts, searching for meaning and purpose.

I didn't feel like I had any place in the world and fought with the despair of wanting to withdraw and stay hidden at home. But God has a plan for me. He has a plan for each of us. With the Holy Spirit to guide and strengthen us, we can carry out that plan and bring Him glory on this earth. If we remain dormant and hidden, the enemy wins, and God's light cannot shine through us to reach the hearts and souls He intends. Every day we are called to step into the world with prayer on our lips, letting the Holy Spirit direct our steps and actions, and giving glory to God in all things:

"You are the light of the world. A town built on a hill cannot be hidden. Neither do people light a lamp and put it under a bowl. Instead, they put it on its stand, and it gives light to everyone in the house. In the same way, let your light shine before others, that they may see your good deeds and glorify your Father in heaven" (Matthew 5:14–16).

DETERMINED TO FIND MY place, and carry out God's will, I prayed for strength and courage. And then finally I was strong enough to go home. Home. Surrounded by a family that loved me made a huge difference in keeping me stable during my recovery. They did not ask for a grand mission or purpose, they only asked for my love and friendship. My nieces and nephews brought so much love and laughter to our family as did my large family with all my brothers and sisters and their spouses. We had many discussions and played many games. They accepted me as I was. Today and now. Let no one doubt the blessing of family and the abundance of life. Every life is a gift of joy and purpose.

One day the thought occurred to me that maybe I could draw. Maybe the talent that had once carved wood could be used with paper and pencil. I sat down with paper and colored pencils. I found I could put the pencil in between my fingers and by moving my arm, I could draw. All the skill I had put into carving and working on teeth could now be put on paper. I decided to sketch a lion, knowing that if I just flicked the pencil across the page and used many lines to create the image instead of relying on a single line I could achieve a complete image. I took a deep breath and calmed my fears. As the lines formed on the page, I relaxed. The lines were crude, and yet as I continued to sketch, the full picture came together and I realized that with this less demanding technique I could create beauty. The thought that I could actually produce something beautiful from my mangled hands gave me a glimmer of hope that this might be a hobby I could invest more time into and be proud of.

The days came and went, overlapping each other. And though I seemed to progress, it was not enough to keep me from being depressed and sad about my current state in life. The daunting idea of the future loomed around me, like a shadow, making me uncertain of where to go, and how to spend my energy. Depression sneaks up on you and then whacks you over the head when you least expect it. Some days, it was obvious what was bugging me, and I could fix it. Other times it was like a dark cloud, and something I just couldn't shake. It crept in when I was having a conversation or interaction, increasing my bad mood and crappy attitude, and yet I didn't know how to fix it. So I just tried to stay out of the way, keep my head down, and spend any of my available energy working out. I gave myself to our Lord and prayed for strength.

God helped me in the most unusual way. A friend of mine called me up, not too long afterward, asking me how

I dealt with depression, mentioning that it didn't make any sense to him. Here he was, able-bodied, able to do the things that he loved, and yet he couldn't shake this feeling of depression. He felt bad reaching out but wanted to know if I had any answer for him. And somewhere in answering him, I realized what God had taught me.

I told him, I might not have a perfect answer, and I might not have the answer that you want to hear, but I believe it is the answer we are all secretly looking for.

Depression sucks, pain sucks, suffering sucks, and yet we have to live with them. The trick is not letting them consume our lives or dictate how we live. The world will tell you that all you need to do is take a fancy pill or buy a product and all of your problems will go away, but that's just not true. Trying to get rid of depression or pain or suffering through any kind of superficial means will often just lead to more pain and suffering, plus an empty wallet. The most important thing with pain, suffering, and depression is accepting it, and then choosing to continue to live despite it. Don't get me wrong, some pain and suffering can be cured, like a cut or disease, but ultimately there will be pain and suffering in this world that we cannot get rid of. We cannot reverse the death of a loved one, we cannot fix the trauma and decisions of the past, but if we can understand that it is a cross that our Lord has given us, then we can bear it well, and continue to live a great life despite it. I shared with him the words of St. Teresa of Avila: "In light of heaven, the worst suffering on earth will be seen as no more than one night in an inconvenient hotel."

Reminding myself of Psalm 126, "Those who sow with tears will reap with songs of joy," I pushed myself to work out, be healthy, take on new hobbies, and reinvent myself.

Ironically, I was following the very advice I had advocated in my thesis so long ago when I was a different man. At the time I took no enjoyment in pushing myself, and everything seemed miserable, but now I find myself looking back on my decisions, and being extremely thankful for what I did, and the future that I've set myself up for. The pain and suffering are not gone, and daily reminders make that apparent, but I am living a full life, and I will continue to do so, until I am finally called home.

One day I received a call from my friend Chris Waker, the fellow survivor of the great tea adventure at Craig Hospital! He told me he was planning on taking a trip up to Yosemite which was only a forty-five-minute drive from my house. He asked if I wanted to meet up. It had been over two years since those days and adventures at Craig, so I happily agreed. The moment I saw him get out of his car, I realized just how much it meant to me to see his improvement and realize my own. We had come so far from struggling to make a cup of tea. We had both grown into our new lives and learned how to adapt our lives to be fulfilling and successful. It was so good to be out there with Chris again, being able to explore the world in a way that we would not have been able to imagine at Craig Hospital so long ago. Poking fun at each other, laughing, joking and reminiscing about old times. It was a beautiful moment, and one that I'll not easily forget. A sign of hope that all was not lost, and the future could indeed be bright and beautiful.

At home, I was and am still blessed and thankful to be surrounded by such loving family members. My three younger brothers are stars for taking on the task of being my caretakers. There have been many long nights and early mornings that involved extreme complications and last-minute medical decisions, but they handled them all like champs. I know I could not have done it without them. The rest of my family very patiently tried to bring me back to life, by subtly engaging me in activities, and trying to find ways to involve me more in family affairs. For now, that meant a lot of board games and a lot of time spent just sitting and talking. I appreciated the effort, and I knew that it was not easy for them either.

Every once in a while, I broke down internally, especially during times when I had typically gathered the family to go play a random sport or construct an obstacle course. Saying goodbye to these interactions is one of the hardest challenges I face and one of the most difficult memories that I really can't get back. It breaks my heart every time, and I just have to close my eyes and offer it up. Sports were such a big part of my life. It is hard to accept that it was all taken in an instant, and unfortunately not something I can easily get back or replace. Whenever those situations come up, the pain of being crippled stings all the more, and I have to step away and do my own thing while they play.

It was during one of these occasions that I reflected on the realization that while we all live together on this earth, when we die, we come face-to-face with God and are judged on our own merits. We are not protected by the pleas or camaraderie of others, but rather only by ourselves, and what was asked of us while we were on this earth.

Then I saw a great white throne and him who was seated on it. The earth and the heavens fled from his presence, and there was no place for them. And I saw the dead, great and small, standing before the throne, and books were opened. Another book was opened, which is the book of life. The dead were judged according to what they had done as recorded in the books. The sea gave up the dead that were in it, and death and Hades gave up the dead that were in them, and each person was judged according to what they had done. Then death and Hades were thrown into the lake of fire. The lake of fire is the second death. Anyone whose name was not found written in the book of life was thrown into the lake of fire (Revelation 20:11–15).

We spend so much time working with or trying to please other people that we often don't have opportunities for self-reflection, and prayerful meditation on what we need to do to improve our lives. We must make sure to prioritize this in our lives, setting aside time every day to reflect on all the good things that God has given us, and all of the things that we have failed to do and need to improve on. We must also use this time to allow God to work on our hearts and speak to us in the silence so that his grace might work through us to better understand his will.

I continued to get stronger and slowly the pain disappeared. It was a great moment when I transitioned back to my manual chair. I started working out, enjoying once again, the feeling of improvement and getting stronger. Although I was still unable to get back the muscles I had lost, I found comfort in the fact that I was at least strengthening the ones that I still had.

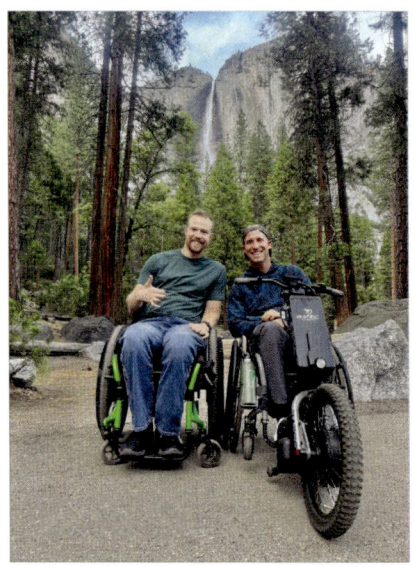

Chris Waker and I in Yosemite

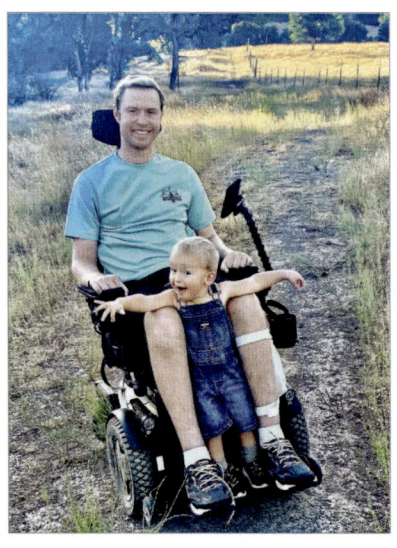

My nephew John and I out back. His big smile and sense of adventure made all the difference.

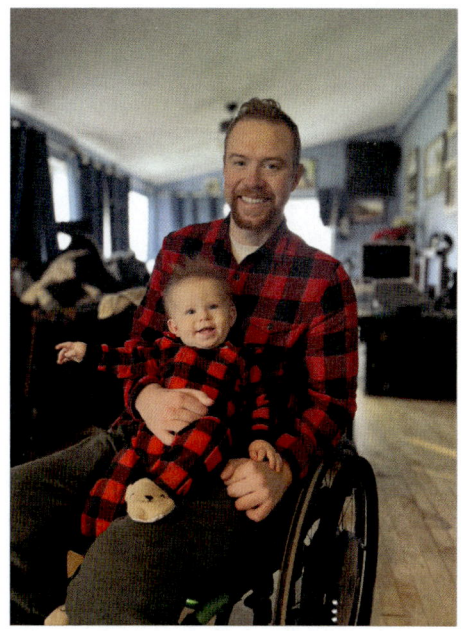

Another of my nephews, my Godson Jerome and I wearing our Christmas plaid.

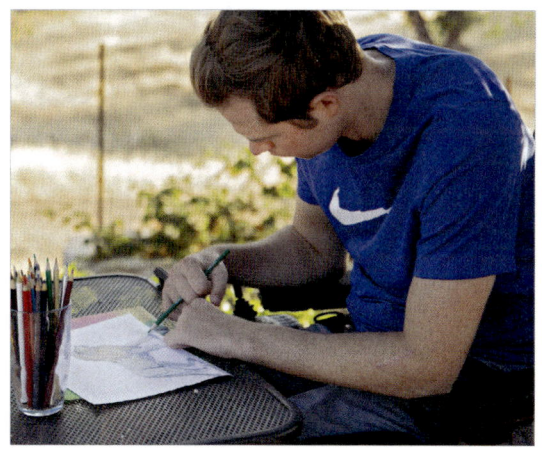

My first attempt at drawing.

CHAPTER 15

PUT ME IN COACH!

Thanksgiving hit, and just like that it had been one year since my accident. A lot of feelings and memories came to mind, but thankfully it also coincided with advent. Advent is the time before Christmas when Christians prepare for the coming of Christ. It is a special period of about four weeks when we dedicate time aside from our daily lives to prepare our hearts and minds for the celebration of Christ's incarnation. During this particular advent, I offered up my sufferings and reflected on God's humility in becoming man. "The Lord himself goes before you and will be with you; He will never leave you nor forsake you. Do not be afraid; do not be discouraged" (Deuteronomy 31:8). These words impressed themselves on my soul as I prepared for Christmas.

As Christmas got closer, everyone worked hard to prepare. All my brothers and sisters were coming home. Christmas Eve was always very special, as we took extra time to pray and reflect on the gospel to grow closer to our Lord as we prepared for the birth of Jesus. Christmas morning finally arrived. We woke up early and went to Mass. We were so excited to spend time with each other, open presents, and hang out. After a beautiful Mass, and saying hi to our friends afterward, we came home, and a cacophony of Christmas traditions began to unfold. Opening presents, eating delectable treats, solving puzzles, and sharing memories. Everyone was full of cheer, full bellies, and, most of all, happy to be with each other. I shed a tear of happiness thanking God for the ability to enjoy Christmas in the way that I had always cherished, compared to a year ago in the hospital room, when life seemed so dark and hopeless.

Christmas came and went, and everyone went their separate ways. As the quiet began to filter back into the house, I contemplated what actually brings us happiness, realizing how little we understand about ourselves. We often encounter moments of joy, but have we taken the time to reflect, and find out what in that moment is actually making us happy. The devil tempts us and tries to convince us that the moment of joy comes from receiving the earthly good, but the reality is much deeper. Much deeper than I even understand. But what I do know is that true joy comes from our participation in God's charity and love. That is why we are so happy when we are with the people that we love. It is why we feel good when we give or show love to others. It is the joy of God's love radiating through us, and our interactions with them. The culmination of all this is our Lord's sacrifice on the cross, pointing the way to the highest form of happiness, which is sacrificial love. Giving of ourselves in a sacrificial manner is so contrary to the way the world has us think, and yet it is the only way that we will ever experience true happiness. It was only after suffering this terrible accident that I truly spent time contemplating it. Notions of how I could ever be happy again after such a tragedy kept running back and forth in my brain, like an itch that you just can't scratch. No matter what I did, it was so hard for me to think that happiness could ever be the same after my accident.

The world certainly tells us that our happiness will be diminished, and the devil plays with our emotions, sending us into depression, believing that is the case. However, it is so far from it. It has now been many years since my accident, and despite what the world would imagine I know that I have found happiness. I have found happiness in my family and friends. I have found happiness in my ability to engage with others intellectually. I have found happiness in serving a purpose, even if the purpose is not what it used to be. But above all else, I have found happiness when learning how to sacrifice myself for others, through prayer and my suffering. The struggle to find happiness comes down to the ability to find love, and more importantly, the love of God in our daily lives. I encourage everyone looking for happiness to look for love, and not selfish love, but sacrificial love. The love our Lord exemplified in his passion and death, dying for our sins. For it is only in that love that we will truly find happiness.

Winter turned to spring, and with the changing seasons came new warmth, and a resolve to get stronger. I once again resumed my workout routine and could feel strength returning to my body. As I got stronger and my health and body began to stabilize, I started signing up for adaptive sports camps, taking on a new challenge of seeing what was possible with adaptive technology. I was both excited and nervous but tempered my expectations as I knew they would be a far cry from what I was used to before my accident. The first one I attended was a summer sports camp in San Diego. Seeing the roster of sports didn't help calm my nerves as along with sailing, fitness, kayaking, and cycling, I saw surfing. Surfing was something that I had always been passionate about and pursued to a great extent through my childhood and then in dental school. Memories of the freedom of being out on the water watching the sunrise and riding the waves into shore, going out to the ocean on a full moon and watching as the ocean turned from a black abyss into shimmering bursts of silver as the waves crashed around my surfboard, filled my mind. There were so many days that I woke up before the crack of dawn and drove out to the beach to catch waves before class started. Surfing has always been a chance for me to escape and find peace and contemplation by myself. It was a big step to return to the ocean in my new paralyzed state, to go back to something that I knew would bear no resemblance to the real thing, to be stripped of that freedom and independence, to be at the mercy of the waves, knowing that with my limited ability to swim I could legitimately drown. Despite my hesitations, I still signed up. The other activities sounded more interesting to me, and I knew pushing myself past my comfort level was where true growth would happen. When the date came, I got in the van with my brother and headed down to San Diego to begin the adventure.

I was excited to arrive in San Diego and meet all the different people, those who had signed up for the adaptive sports as well as all the many men and women making this happen. We were given a schedule, and the activity I expected to be the most boring was sailing. Sailing was something that I did not have a lot of prior experience with, and so my expectations coming into it were fairly minimal. I expected nothing more than sitting on the boat while it moved through the water. I joked with my family that I expected to be tied to the mast, like the classic movie that we had watched as a kid called *What About Bob*. But the reality of what transpired could not be further from my expectations.

We started off in a classroom setting going over all the details of the boats and instructions, and although I had my doubts about how important the information would be for me or what my role would be on the boat, I still paid attention and tried to learn. When it finally came time for us to approach the boat and get on it, they asked if I wanted to be in the captain's position and lead the boat around the bay. I was honored and appreciated the responsibility, but that was only half of it. They put me in the chair with the rudder, the steering wheel of the boat, and it was my responsibility to direct us around the ocean. My brain started firing on all cylinders as I realized not only that this was going to be a challenge, but also a challenge that I could handle. I began calling out orders to change the tightness of the lines and directing the ship with the wind patterns to maximize our speed and collect the tokens that were placed around the bay for the competition. I had never felt so empowered from something that I had almost written off. My capabilities were tested both intellectually and physically as I fought the strong pull of the ocean and kept a sturdy heading across the water. By the time it was over, I almost didn't want to get off. It felt so good to not feel limited by my disability and really be able to push my limits. It was a complete success, and our team placed first. It also really opened up my eyes to how much adaptive sports and events can change the way that we look at things.

I wish that I could say the same about surfing. Surfing was brutally hard to do, both on a physical and emotional level. Knowing that I did not have the strength or ability to paddle out on my own and that I could not stand or even kneel to ride the wave in, it was hard to accept that I would need to rely on someone else to balance my surfboard as others pushed me into the shore. It was hard to come face-to-face with just how different my life was now. Everything that I had loved about the sport was gone, and I had to acknowledge it. It was hard going back to something that reminded me so closely of all that I had before. That loss was a wound that cut deep and brought with it a wave of sorrow and sadness for what would never be again. I put on a smile for everyone that was there, thankful for their work. I understood that it was not only my time, but the time and energy of so many dedicated volunteers, coaches, and therapists, doing their best to help us enjoy what we could in this new world of ours. I knew others got enjoyment from it, but that sport was not for me; it hit too close to home and I could not even recognize it for what it was.

The whole experience helped me learn a valuable lesson. I realized that with traumatic and life altering events like mine, the only solution was to reinvent myself. I had to go back to the drawing board and look for new experiences to try, like sailing. It was important for me to learn something without a comparison to how it was before. By doing this, I was able to appreciate exciting new opportunities and activities with fresh eyes and appreciate doing them to the extent I could without feeling any lack. I encourage everyone in any similar situation to look at life with fresh eyes and take on new challenges that do not constantly leave you thinking about what you had before. I have found this to be very helpful in coping with my injury and growing from it. Now don't get me wrong, there are so many things that I do now that I also did before my accident, but I make a point to try many new things that I have never done before, in order to help develop a new notion of who I am.

I arrived home from the event, and life carried on as normal for the next couple of weeks, but then one day when I was working out, I suddenly started hacking up some bloody phlegm. At first, I thought nothing of it, as it was just a little bit of blood, probably nothing to be worried about. But it kept happening throughout the day, and for the next several days. I continued to have blood in my mucus, and the coughing and hacking were getting worse. I was convinced that it was just something to do with the weather, and not a serious problem. My mom was worried and so we did some research. We learned that there was a small chance it could be a blood clot. We decided that it was best for my mom to take me to the emergency room. They checked my blood levels, and something seemed off, but they said they needed to do a CAT scan to figure out more. I got into the machine with swirling lights and loud sounds and waited to hear the results. After the test was done, I went to the waiting room where we sat patiently to hear what was going on. The doctor came back in disbelief.

"I honestly can't believe you're still alive," he said. "You have multiple pulmonary embolisms. Blood clots in the lungs. Typically, people can die from just one, but you have over twenty."

He told me that they seemed small enough not to obstruct the arteries but were causing damage to my lungs. Immediately they sent me to the VA hospital in Palo Alto for further treatment. I barely had time to say goodbye before the ambulance picked me up and I was escorted away. I said goodbye, not knowing if this would be my last. I arrived at the hospital just around midnight, and I was immediately put on heavy IV anticoagulants to help break up the clots in my lungs and ensure that I didn't die.

The treatment seemed to be working, and I was thankful, once again, to narrowly escape death. I reflected on how many times I had been so close to death. And I knew that since I wasn't dead yet, God must have some greater plans for me. I just hoped they didn't include getting sick every couple of months with a life-threatening condition. After about a week of closely monitored treatment and some post-op instructions for the blood thinner, I was in good enough shape to head home and resume my life. Even after returning home, it was hard to get over the idea that another life-threatening illness could possibly be looming right around the corner. Every time I seemed to make progress, I felt like it was erased by sickness and recovery. Even though I knew God had a greater plan for me, it was hard for me to see where I fit into that picture. Every time I felt like I was getting to the point where I could contribute, I was knocked back again.

I had a conversation with my spiritual director, a great priest who agreed to help guide my spiritual life. I explained the difficulty I'd had, feeling like I couldn't do anything, feeling like I was on the sidelines, and I so badly wanted to play in the game. What he said next stayed with me forever: "You are not on the sidelines; you are the one playing the game. We are the ones on the sidelines, cheering you on through our prayers."

He continued, "The real battle is not a battle of our physical accomplishment, but rather the spiritual battle that takes place in our soul. Your physical suffering and limitations bring you that much closer to God and that much deeper into the spiritual battlefield. God has chosen you as a warrior to fight on the front lines for the spiritual good of others. Pray to God for the strength to take on your role and suffer and pray for the cross of Christ."

I think back to those words and continually resubmit myself to God's will. "I am your soldier, Lord; I am here to serve you in any way that I can." Some days that prayer is hard to say and even harder to understand, but it bolsters my spirit to pray harder and offer up my suffering for God's will.

I very much felt the need to be productive during the day, and so I prayed about what I could do. Dental school was a distant and painful memory and hard to recollect without feeling remorse for what was gone. Everything that my life seemed to culminate in had been stripped from me before my eyes, never to be seen again. However, many people in the dental field were gracious enough to help connect me to the representatives at the California Dental Association. They reached out to me with an offer to work with students, helping them to transition from being students to practicing dentists. The offer felt like a two-edged sword; on the one hand I was more than thankful for an opportunity to pursue a job in the field that I loved so much, but on the other hand, it was hard to be so close to dentistry and know that I would never be a dentist. I knew it would be an emotional roller-coaster, but I graciously accepted the offer, and I was thankful for the opportunity to get back into the workforce.

I took on the job of student programs consultant, helping work with the student program team to lead students through dental school and beyond. I was able to provide them with the resources they needed to have a successful career and mitigate the difficulties that would arise along the way. Although my work was mostly in the background, it felt good to be able to help the students.

I learned the basics of what we were trying to do and took off, enjoying the ability to add a unique perspective to the team by being so close in age to the students. Work became part of my daily routine, as I got up each morning, had breakfast, did my work, worked out, hung out with my brothers, had dinner, and went to bed. I enjoyed this aspect of normality, having my day filled with meaningful tasks, and ways to improve myself. There was still more that I needed to accomplish in the future, but for right now, it gave me satisfaction to know that I was doing good.

Going around the grocery store one day, I was caught off guard when someone, seeing how much progress I'd made since the accident, said, "What a miracle, God is good." These words struck me hard, because I immediately thought it wrong to give all the credit to God, when I was the one who had worked so hard and suffered so much to get where I was. I was the one pushing myself to overcome obstacles and fighting to adapt. Where was God when I needed a miracle to be cured, where was he when I was struggling to get through the day? Where was he when my muscles were failing, and where was he during all of my pain?

As I pondered this, I thought back to when my spinal cord had a cyst growing in it, and every day my energy dwindled and my ability to do anything disappeared. I told a priest that all I wanted to do was be able to help myself get better, and that it wasn't fair that God had taken away even the ability to help myself.

And then it hit me: God wanted me to know that even my ability to make myself better is a gift from him. I might've had a hand in my progress, but truly all of it is a gift from God and a miracle that I am able to accomplish it. All of my success and accomplishments, all that I have overcome truly is a miracle, and a gift from God.

So, I challenge you to think about what you are most proud of—the things you have poured your time, energy, and heart into. Reflect on your greatest achievements and the moments when hard work finally paid off. Then recognize this truth: none of it was accomplished by your strength alone. Every ability, every opportunity, and every success is a gift from God. Without His grace, we have nothing; however with it, all things become possible.

> "Non nobis Domine, non nobis,
> sed nomini tuo da gloriam."
> Not to us Lord, not to us,
> but to thy name let the glory be given.

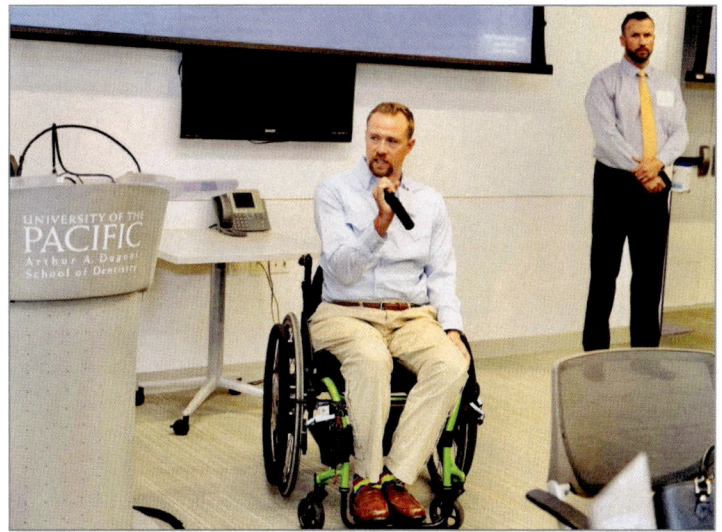

Giving a speech for the CDA

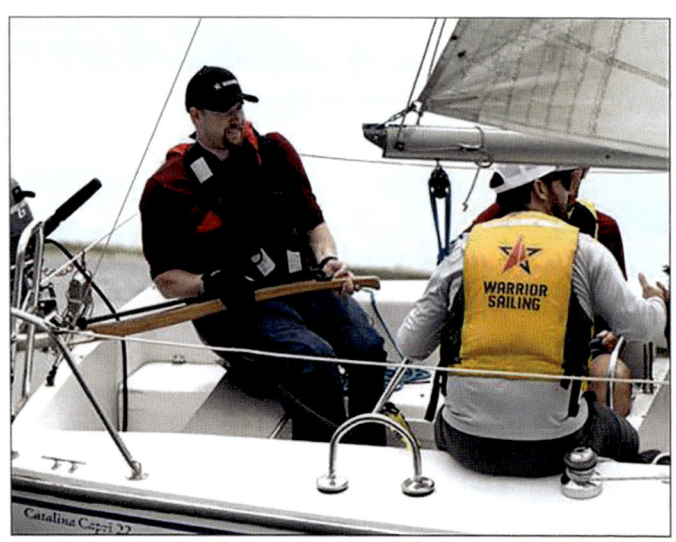

Sailing!

CHAPTER 16

ALL FOR HIM

As I started to get stronger and more independent in my day-to-day functions, and set up a life for myself, I began to think about getting the second planned surgery for my hands. This would involve a tendon transfer. The surgery would be more involved than the first one and would involve cutting tendons from working muscles within my arm and reattaching them to a group of finger muscles in my hand. These additional surgeries would help bring back some more functionality to my hands. They would not allow my fingers to move independently of one another, but they would allow my fingers to close all at once and provide me with grip and more independence in my daily life. I knew that even with this increasing function, I would still be limited, but my capabilities would be far greater. I talked to the doctors about the surgeries, and they explained that there was about four months recovery time for each hand before I would be able to fully take advantage of it. I knew that eight months would set me back a great deal when it came to working out and living my life, but I also knew that this surgery would increase the threshold of what I was able to do in the future. I thought and prayed about it and realized that the best time to do it was now, when I was young and relatively healthy, so there were fewer chances for complications and more time to recover. I explained to them that if we were going to do them, I would like to do them back-to-back so as to minimize any downtime and maximize my future time. They agreed and scheduled the first one at the end of September. I got together with some of my good friends for one last hurrah before I bit the bullet and dove headfirst into what I knew would be a very long and hard eight months.

I headed back to the hospital preparing for the worst, and after several tests to make sure my heart was in good condition, I finally headed into surgery. The surgery was almost eight hours, and I woke up, groggy and sore, pain radiating through my arm down to my fingers. I tried to sleep, knowing that it would be helpful for my recovery. However, with all of the meds, it was hard for my body to find deep sleep. Instead, I simply passed in and out of consciousness, like some kind of discordant dream. Deep in the recesses of my mind, I prayed, offering up my suffering, praying for the strength to persevere. My body spasmed in response to the surgery, sending new aching pains shooting down my arm. I recited the words from scripture, "this too will pass." That night was one of the worst of my life. I was unable to sleep, as the pain got worse and worse. I tried to subdue it with medication, and yet each time, the pain threshold was broken through. I didn't sleep and could only call out for help when the pain became too much. I lay in the dark, praying for the moment when I would see sunlight and this night from hell would be over. I kept battling, and eventually the rays of golden sunlight filtered into my room, bringing with them warmth and hope for a new day. I thanked God for the fact that my room faced the sun, thinking back to my days in the ICU when for forty days I never saw the sun.

They changed up my pain medication, and for the first time, I actually felt relief. It amazed me how pain medication worked. Part of me wondered if there is some lack of strength in my character that kept me from just accepting the pain and offering it up for the salvation of souls. After all, Christ didn't get pain medication for his suffering. So many of the saints did not take or get pain medication. I know that it is good for me to take pain medication to get better, and yet I can't help but wonder. Removing the pain makes the circumstances so much easier to deal with. I trusted that God had put me in the situation to experience some pain without having to bear all of it. I have no doubt that God could give me pain without any cure or aid if he really wanted to. I was thankful for the break from suffering, and the ability to sleep peacefully.

The rest of the week was all recovery and pain management. When I was finally back in my chair, and the pain was manageable enough, I headed home for the rest of my recovery and the beginning of my rehab. I knew that patience and the waiting was the hardest part. At this point, I'd gotten used to working and moving in my manual chair; however, because one of my arms was out of commission for the next several months I had to go back into my power chair where I could control it with only one arm. The power chair felt stifling and scary. It was all part of the recovery, but it was one part that I didn't look forward to. My manual chair felt like an extension of my body, responding to the tactile push of my arms and force of my movements. Whereas the power chair felt very disconnected, moving around with just the flick of my wrist, having so much power and no ability to determine the force applied in my movements. This made it terrifying to be around little kids as there was no tactile feedback if I was running into them. I felt distanced from the world, almost as if I was driving a car just to get from my bedroom to the dining-room table.

The only consolation that I had from being in the power chair was that it had the ability to lean back, so tilting it and taking a nap became my new favorite part of the day. The chair took no exertion to operate, and so it allowed me to focus primarily on recovering and not expending my energy just moving around. It was very difficult to do everything with one hand. So many of my daily interactions involved both hands. All my downtime was spent with audiobooks and TV shows, while I also had plenty of room for naps in the middle of the day.

After a couple of weeks, my energy level started to return, and I went back to work. I was excited to put my intellect to use while my hand recovered. However, despite being back at work, the lack of independence and difficulty with simple tasks started to catch up with me, and I became more irritable to those around me. I had a short fuse and often took out my irritability on them with harsh criticisms or angry words.

How often in our life are we ruled by our emotions? We don't always realize how prevalent a role they play in our daily actions and choices; however, more often than not, they dictate our every action. If we are feeling happy, then we happily engage with others; if we are feeling angry or sad, then we usually let everyone know it or bury it deep inside. It is important to acknowledge our own emotions but not let them control us. For if we love only when we feel like it, it merits us nothing. "If you love those who love you, what credit is that to you? For even sinners love those who love them" (Luke 6:32).

True charity comes about when we are tasked with acting contrary to our emotions and different from how we feel. This might be in the form of showing love to someone we don't feel love for or smiling and having a friendly conversation with someone even when we're having a bad day. We must constantly push ourselves to look beyond our own emotions and act out of the charity in our hearts. Integrity is how we act when no one is looking. Charity is how we act when we don't feel like it. "Love your enemies, do good, and lend, expecting nothing in return. Your reward will be great, and you will be children of the Most High" (Luke 6:36).

How easy it is to say these words, and yet how difficult it is to live by them. Especially since my accident, I have struggled with this more than ever before. It takes so much strength to push beyond my feelings and engage with others in a positive way. This task is by no means easy, but it is necessary if we wish to enter into salvation. For it is only when we are put to the test that we can be truly purified.

After two months of what seemed like an eternity of recovering, my hand was finally ready to start being used again. At first it felt stiff and rigid, making it too difficult to do even the simplest tasks. My brain slowly started to work out the kinks with the new muscles, and as I began therapy, it became apparent how much of a difference this was already making in my life. The ability to grab and pick things up was a monumental change. The movements were awkward, and very limited in functionality, but just as Jesus multiplied the loaves and fishes, so I could take this humble movement and turn it into something great.

Just as God planted the seed of faith and it grew into a mighty oak tree, the spark of creativity helped me to realize the potential of this newfound strength. The more I did with my hand, the easier the movements became. Although there were definitely limits, I was happy to see my body adapting and willing to take on new challenges. A lot of my daily tasks became easier, and I found that I was able to do things more efficiently, and with more confidence. As I got closer to the three-month mark, I began talking with the doctors about doing the other hand. I knew that the longer I waited the harder it would be to go into surgery again, so I committed to starting surgery in the next two weeks.

Before I knew it, the day was here, I said goodbye to my family as I shuttled into the car and was transported back to the hospital. It was hard going back a second time, knowing that I was getting the same surgery, knowing that I would experience the same pains, knowing that I would experience the same weaknesses. PTSD crept into my mind and caused me great anxiety, so many steps were similar that I could not help my brain from panicking. I turned to God for strength and didn't let my emotions take control of me; instead, I focused on completing the task at hand each day, not letting other thoughts get in the way of my recovery. The surgery went well, and once again I was lying in bed, holding my breath for fear that if I let it go, I would have to come face-to-face with the reality of how long my recovery would be.

Surprisingly, the pain was not nearly as bad this time around. I suspected a big part of that had to do with the fact that I had less sensation in this arm, so it made sense that I wouldn't feel as much pain. After only about a week, I found myself back at home, waiting for my hand to heal in the splint while I tried to manage everything with my offhand. This in and of itself wasn't so bad, although it took quite a bit of getting used to, especially eating, brushing my teeth, and using my computer.

However, after a couple of weeks, the déjà vu of my recovery process made time slow to a crawl, it made everything that much harder to bear. I now felt like I'd been in recovery for six months rather than two weeks, because so many of the memories blended together. However, because the pain was much easier to manage this time, it became a game of patience more than anything else.

While my hand slowly healed, I began to plan events in my future. It felt good being able to focus on what life had in store, rather than just surviving the next surgery. I began writing this book, started making plans to learn how to drive and get an adaptive vehicle, and signed up for two separate sports clinics to help expand my knowledge of what I could do and what was available to me. Additionally, I started taking up chess, finding it stimulating for my brain and giving me some fun competition while I recovered. The competition was good for my soul, especially since I had always been an overachiever and had a competitive spirit, so finding a way to challenge my mind without taxing my body was a blessing. I continued to draw and was pleased to see my talent grow and manifest itself. Filled with love for our crucified Lord, I drew a sketch of Christ's face as he turned to his father and said, "Into your hands I commend my spirit." I gave it to my father because of how much his strength and faith have always inspired me and helped me to go forward when I did not think I could. In another moment of prayer, I was inspired to draw the gentle features of Our Lady, her eyes lifted toward heaven in contemplation.

I sketched her as a birthday gift to my mother, because her quiet strength, tender love, and steadfast faith have always reminded me of the Virgin Mary's strength and character.

In the past, I often got caught up with the thought that everything I did needed to be exceptional or perfect. Oftentimes I found myself shying away from doing something because I did not think that I would excel at it. Most recently, I felt this way about writing this book, trying to determine whether it was worth writing when I often struggle with what to say, and don't always have a deep inspiration to pull from. I have been contemplating this for the last year and have come to two conclusions. The first is that we cannot give up on something just because it's hard or we're not great at it. It's funny how this is such a simple concept that we're taught over and over again, and yet how often every single day we choose to avoid things that we struggle with, or things that don't come naturally to us. The second conclusion is that we all have natural abilities and talents that God has given us, and we owe it to him to make the most of them. "Like good stewards of the manifold grace of God, serve one another with whatever gift each of you has received" (1 Peter 4:10). One conclusion says we have to work on what we struggle with, while the other says we have to do what comes naturally to us. While these seem conflicting, they're not mutually exclusive. In fact, some of our gifts are not made manifest until we put in the hard work. So while writing might not come easily to me, I owe it to God to put in the hard work and let him do the rest. "I can do all things through him who strengthens me" (Philippians 4:13).

I challenge each and every one of you to pursue something that seems difficult to you, but that you feel called to do. Put in the time and the hard work, and if it is something that you were meant to do, God will take care of the rest. If you are not meant to follow that path, God will close it for you and open a new one.

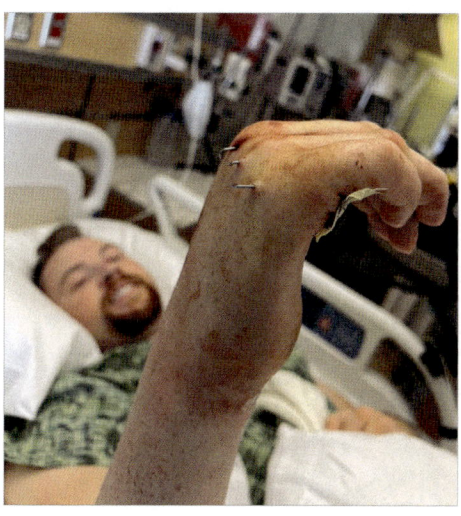

Just after my tendon surgery. Notice the pins coming out of my hand. I joked that I looked like a wolverine.

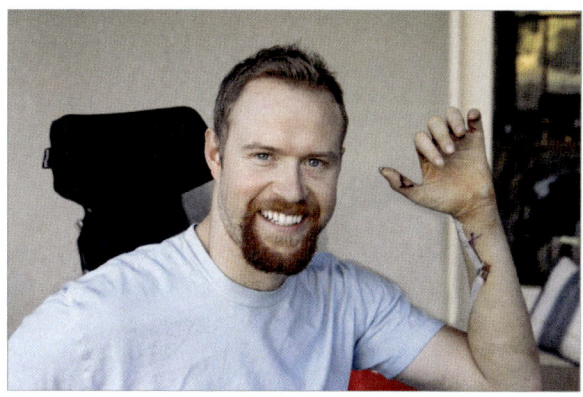

The impressive wound in my hands and forearm after the surgery.

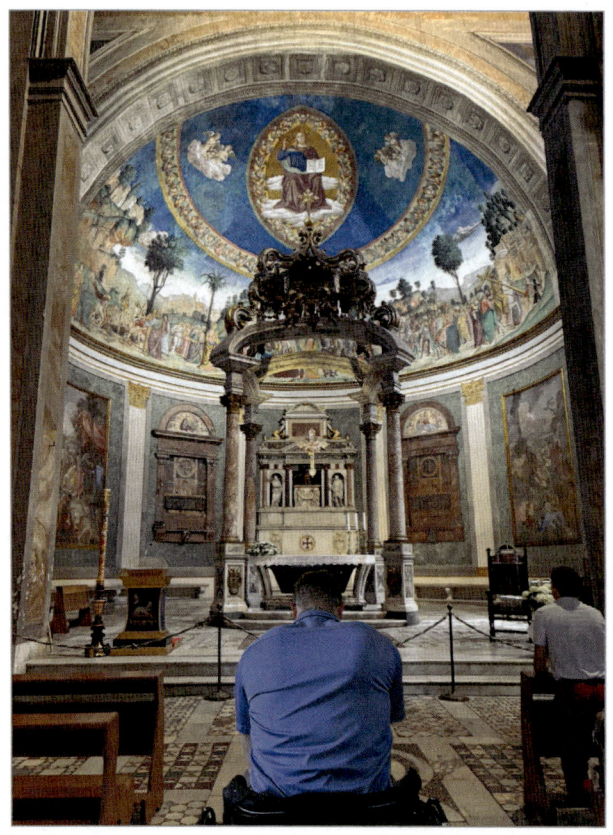

Adoring our Lord in a church in Italy

Pushing Through the Pain

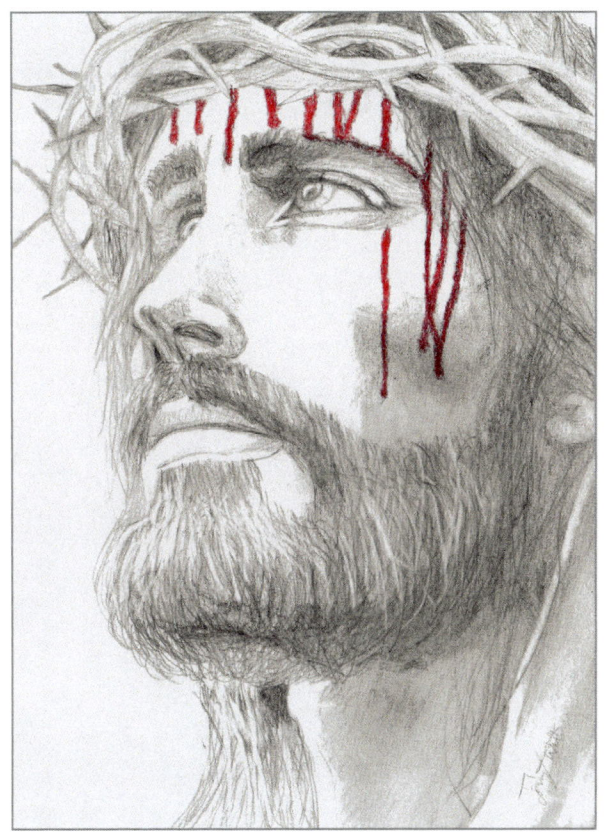

My drawing of our Lord crying out to His Father

Conclusion

PAIN HAS BEEN MY constant companion—sometimes a quiet shadow, sometimes a storm at full force. It has lingered at the edges of nearly every chapter of my life, whispering that I couldn't go on, daring me to quit, taunting me with everything I had lost. Yet pain has also been my teacher. It has forced me to dig deeper than I thought possible, to reach for strength I did not have on my own, and to rely completely on our Father who never abandons his children.

The world tells us to run from pain. We numb it with pills, drown it in distraction, hide it behind carefully curated images, or pretend it doesn't exist. The message is always the same: if you hurt, something is wrong with you—fix it fast, and don't let anyone see the cracks. I lived that way before my accident, but when my injury came, there was no quick fix. No product or mindset could erase the reality of what had happened to me. It was in that place of helplessness that I discovered the truth: avoiding pain may bring temporary comfort, but it robs us of the growth, wisdom, and intimacy with God that only comes when we face it head-on.

The world says comfort is the goal; Christ says the cross is the path. The world says chase the life you want; Christ says follow me, even when the way is hard. I could not have understood this if all my prayers had been answered with ease. Pain taught me that victory is not found in escaping hardship, but in enduring it—and not by my strength, but by his.

Suffering is inescapable in this life. The question is not if the cross will come, but when it does, how we will carry it. We can drag it in resentment, letting it bruise and weigh us down, or we can lift it with Christ, letting his strength become our own. When we choose to carry our cross with love, it changes everything. What once felt like a prison becomes a passageway. The burden that threatens to crush us becomes the very thing that draws us closer to the heart of Christ, where suffering is transformed into an offering—a sharing in the saving work of the cross.

I wish I could say I have mastered this, that I handle every setback with perfect trust. The truth is, I still have a long way to go. There are days when frustration wins, when I grow impatient with my limitations and when I forget to pray before acting. This injury has revealed not only the weakness of my body, but the weakness of my heart in trusting God fully.

And yet, every time I reach the end of myself, God carries me. His strength pushes me when mine is gone—sometimes through a clear answer to prayer, but more often through quiet, steady nudges: one more therapy repetition when I want to quit, one conversation I'd rather avoid, one morning choosing to get up when staying in bed would be easier. Each push matters. Each one moves me forward, even when progress is hard to see.

Pushing through pain does not mean ignoring it. It means facing it, feeling its weight, and still moving toward Christ who gives hope. It means clinging to his promises so deeply that even without seeing the end, you take the next push forward. Sometimes that push gains ground;

other times it simply holds your position so you don't lose what you've fought for. But even holding your ground with him is a victory.

If you are facing pain—whether visible or hidden—know this: your struggle is real, but so is your strength in Christ. The path may be long, the slope steep, and your arms tired, but you are not in this alone. Keep pushing forward, one turn of the wheels at a time. One day, you will look back from the summit and realize that every push, every sorrow, every moment you thought you couldn't move another inch was carrying you toward something far greater than you imagined.

And when you reach that summit, the view will take your breath away—not because the climb was easy, but because of who climbed it with you. You will see that every step was taken with our Lord, making your burden lighter and giving you strength when you had none left. You will see the faces of those who came to know Love because you refused to quit, and you will know that from the first page of your story to the last, Christ was shaping you for this triumph. Then you will hear him say, "Well done, my good and faithful servant." And in that moment, you will know without a doubt—it was worth it.

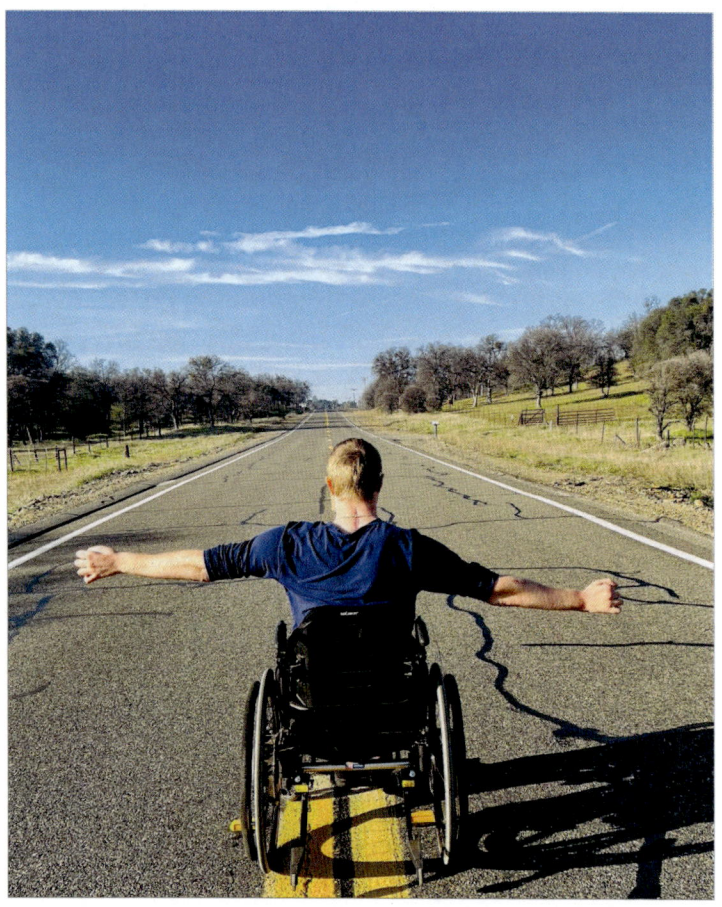

On the open road near our home

Made in the USA
Coppell, TX
12 February 2026

71074917R00117